THE PSYCHOMATRIX

THE PSYCHOMATRIX
A Deeper Understanding
of Our Relationship with Pain

Doreen M. Francis

KARNAC

First published in 2015 by
Karnac Books Ltd
118 Finchley Road
London NW3 5HT

British Library Cataloguing in Publication Data

A C.I.P. for this book is available from the British Library

ISBN-13: 978-1-78220-318-6

Typeset by V Publishing Solutions Pvt Ltd., Chennai, India

Printed in Great Britain

www.karnacbooks.com

To my sons, Andrew and Peter, who allowed me to run away, grow up, and face my pain just enough to be inspired to fulfil my fantasy of writing this book—and this is only the beginning …

AMDG

Happiness is a by-product of meaning as pleasure is a by-product of pain, therefore to find meaning one must suffer one's pain to know the other …

CONTENTS

INTRODUCTION

A cold in the head causes less suffering than an idea.

—*Jules Renard*, 1864–1910

The aim of this book is to argue that it is not pain, as such, but the relationship of the subject to (his) pain, which is most significant to his processes of life.

The first thing that comes to mind when we hear the word pain is *physical pain*. The second thought is usually about psychological or emotional pain, but only after some deliberation. Historically, research has primarily focused on physical pain and pain processing. Scientists such as Melzack and Wall (1965) developed the most recent theories about the neurological processing of pain, which has allowed research to progress into other aspects of pain, mainly into the psychological impact and the significance of the correlations between physical and psychological pain. However, the main premise of pain research continues to be neurological and not psychological. The paradigm that "pain" must have a neurological cause is a challenging one to surmount as those, for example with "chronic pain", seek a solution primarily within the physical when it has been evidenced through research (Gamsa, 1994) that much "chronic pain" is situated in an individual's psychological and emotional dimensions.

Continuing the research that he and Wall began in the 1960s, Melzack (1993) developed the concept of the neuromatrix that situated pain processing in the brain. Having a background in psychology it was inevitable that Melzack also gave significant credence to the impact of an individual's psychological and emotional environment.

Melzack and Wall (1996) proposed that pain is not simply a function that relays a message that there is damage to the body, but that there is also the impact of our previous experiences that influence the amount and quality of the pain we feel. Our ability to understand the causes of our pain, and to grasp the consequences, also influences our subjective experience of pain. In the same source, Melzack explains that "even the culture in which we have been brought up plays an essential role in how we feel and respond to pain" (p. 15).

Since it is pain that establishes its presence first in the subject's life (i.e., loss) I would argue that it is pain that defines his identity. The pursuit of pleasure to avoid *being in* pain is unachievable, so keeps one in a perverse cycle of repetitive behaviour. It is for this reason that the subject must become aware of and realise the need to establish his relationship with his *pain*.

In order to evidence my theory I will examine Freud's psychosexual theory of development, including his seminal work and his conceptualisations in *A Project for a Scientific Psychology* (1950a) and Melzack's theory of the neuromatrix as developed in the 1990s following his and Wall's influential research on pain and pain processing.

This study mainly concentrates on a psychoanalytic model of pain, the main focus of which is Freudian. However, I would also like to acknowledge Lacan's seminal contributions to contemporary psychoanalytic discussion and most notably post-Freudian developments. It would behove me, *en passant*, to give credence to the Lacanian notion of *jouissance*, which is apposite to my inquiry and which provides some seminal insights of this investigation. *Jouissance* with its sexual etymology connotes more than mere enjoyment but, rather, the pleasure inherent in pain and the pain of too much pleasure. Tickling and sexual climax would be two concrete examples that testify to the impossibility of satisfaction. Even here, we see the emotive relational sphere being accessed within one's desire for the perfect pleasure.

According to Professor Fry's (2009) Yale University lecture on Lacanian theory, it seems that Lacan's narrative on desire is the notion of a sustaining of desire which goes through a series of detours which result in a continuation of desire, resulting in an *ending* that may correspond to what Freud referred to as the *desire* of the subject to die in its own way without external pressure. We may fulfil our needs (such as physical hunger); however, desire (fulfilling an emotional and psychological need) is an entirely different matter.

The *pain* I wish to discuss in my book is this desire which Freud speaks of and which Lacan expands upon. Desire is an interminable entity during the state and circumstance of human living. At the moment of loss, the subject embarks upon a journey of desire. In other words he sets out to find that piece of the puzzle which will fit exactly and so perfectly into the space or lack, so that the unity or whole would be as before, without evidence of the loss—the perfect pleasure, that which is beyond the pain of desire.

The complexity it seems lies in the subject's knowledge—"symbolic" knowledge, which expresses the subject's desire and lives in the unconscious and "imaginary" knowledge, which is narcissistic and a false sense of the self and ego. "Imaginary knowledge" is knowledge that acts as a barrier to "symbolic knowledge", which expresses the desire of the subject and which is considered a form of jouissance (Evans, 2006 p. 94). According to Mills (2003), Lacan's theory of "imaginary knowledge" is that it is a "paranoiac knowledge" and postulates that:

> Developmentally, knowledge is paranoiac because it is acquired through our *imaginary* relation to the other as a primordial misidentification or illusory self-recognition of autonomy, control, and mastery, thus leading to persecutory anxiety and self-alienation. Secondarily, through the *symbolic* structures of language and speech, desire is foisted upon us as a foreboding demand threatening to invade and destroy our uniquely subjective inner experiences. And finally, the process of knowing itself is paranoiac because it horrifically confronts the *real*, namely, the unknown. [...] paranoiac knowledge manifests itself as the desire not to know. (p. 30)

As Kierkegaard (Hong & Hong, 2000) has expressed, that anxiety is fear of the known as well as the unknown. The problem, I suggest, is this very "desire not to know". The mere notion of this is what triggers the pursuit of this knowledge. Albeit the pursuit takes many "detours" (Fry, 2009) and forms, it continues throughout life. The interminable pursuit evidences the existence of a lack and its desire, within the unconscious of the subject. This knowledge, I argue, presumes a *relationship* between the subject and his pain, pain that is at the heart of desire. The subject's *relationship* to his pain then, is his desire to find pleasure or more correctly, to pursue pleasure in spite of his knowledge.

I would suggest that the behaviours that accompany such pursuit would fall into the realm of what, in psychoanalytic terms, would be categorised as neurosis, particularly as I consider the case samples which I have chosen to use in my book. The defence mechanisms which one employs to reach the "perfect" pleasure or satisfaction and avoid pain are often mechanisms that bring one pain, which in turn dictates the processes to achieving this aim. They also dictate the amount of pain one needs in order to reach this end. As I consider the subject matter of my book it is clear that a thread that may run subtly through it is a suggestion that we are obsessed with our obsessions to escape our pain—actually I propose that we are obsessed with our pain and how to make it provide us with the ultimate pleasure that we seek. This as we know brings us dangerously close to annihilation and into the realm of the impossibility of desire and *jouissance* (Lacan, 1992).

Miller (2011) alludes to this when he reminds us of Freud's mention in the case of *Dora* that "[o]f all the clinical pictures which we meet with, in clinical medicine, it is the phenomena of intoxication and abstinence in connection with the use of certain chronic poisons that most closely resemble the psychoneuroses" (Freud, 1905e).

What is most significant to this book is Miller's comment in this same paragraph that "upon further reflection, we are reminded that neurotic symptoms provide satisfactions similar to those provided by intoxicating and addictive substances" (2011, p. 164).

Therefore, it may be that the subject is addicted to the effects—highs and lows—of his choice of intoxicant. We can clearly see this in Freud's research in *The Cocaine Papers* (1963). Loose (2011) draws on this research on cocaine and writes that "the decisive factor regarding the effect of cocaine, is something in the psyche of the user" in that it has an indirect effect on the body "via a psychic variable". And, therefore, addiction is influenced by something within the individual (p. 4).

As in any relational situation, one is inevitably confronted with answering the question of what it means to have a "connection" with the other, in this case pain. Part and parcel of this connection is fear of loss and fulfilment of desire. Pain dictates pleasure—without pain, one knows nothing of pleasure. If we began our lives not knowing the pain of loss, there would be no need to seek to fulfil that loss and reunite with the lost object. It is interesting that when we look at the ways in which society is travelling, each individual seems to be involved in searching to fill some feeling of emptiness or such—in behaviour such as obsessive shopping, gambling, drug addiction and breakdowns in the family unit, divorce, homelessness, child abuse, chronic pain, war and its products, such as being limbless and post-traumatic stress disorders. It can be argued that it is all in the service of finding something to fill the void or lack. As Loose (2011) has suggested, in our society today there is a sense that *jouissance* and pleasure have become so that it is one's "duty", or as I would understand, one's *right* to have this. He explains that it appears as if "[w]e have to enjoy ourselves because we have at our disposal and in abundance all the products (such as drugs and alcohol) and gadgets with which to do it" (p. 3).

And therefore, we stop at nothing to reach our objective. Loose argues that "the push to find solutions outside oneself for one's problems and discontents, as well as the duty of enjoyment in recent times, fuel the *addictification* of our society" (ibid.).

Here I define *pain* as a conglomerate (or collection) of experiences from the world (reality) we perceive around us, shrouded in social constructs, laws, meanings, and desires. When what is real (the materiality of ourselves and our misperceptions) confronts us, it is disruptive and painful (Felluga, 2011). These experiences are thus imprinted on the unconscious. Within these experiences lies what is real and it is with this *real* that the subject must acquaint him or her *self*. It is this (acquaintance) relationship that is the *real reality* that establishes identity and impacts on the subject's existence.

Outline of this book

Chapter One will examine the definition and historical perspective of pain. It will also examine the present day notion of pain (from a neurological perspective) as a vital sign of (human) life as it will serve as a further introduction to my theory of the subject-pain relationship.

In Chapter Two I will discuss Freud's *A Project for a Scientific Psychology* (1950a) and examine its explanation of the neurological processes of pain and their physical and psychological impacts. This will also provide an understanding of memory, motive, and perception, and Freud's definition of pain—physical as well as emotional. The next section will be an explanation of Melzack and Wall's neurological definition of pain and its psychological and emotional correlations. This will lead to a comparison of Melzack's theory of the neuromatrix and Freud's neurological theory outlined in his *Project*.

Chapter Three will further discuss my theory of the psychomatrix, which I have derived from Freud's explanation in his *Project* as well as Melzack's theory of the neuromatrix.

I will also discuss the theory of pain from Freud's psychoanalytic perspective and in so doing I will endeavour to further explain the significance of my concept of the psychomatrix and the subject-pain relationship. Freud's research efforts in his *Project* influenced his subsequent work and I argue that all his theories and concepts spring from his desire to identify human pain, its processes, and its purpose. He began from a neurological premise that soon implicated the psychological; so much so that all his subsequent work gave primacy to the human psyche and its cognitive and behavioural manifestations.

I will work toward establishing definitions of subject, relationship, identity, existence, and pain in order to construct a frame of reference that will further inform my book.

Chapter Four will begin the discussion and analyses of case scenarios to further evidence my thesis. The first case scenario, presented in this chapter, will be that of the phantom limb syndrome. The phantom limb syndrome, as investigated by Melzack (1993, 2006) and Ramachandran (1998), is pain that exists in a part of the body, particularly a limb, which no longer exists—for example, a limb which has been amputated due to a disease or accident. The mind is fixated on the part of the body that no longer exists, suffering its loss and desiring to fill the empty space—as we have heard tell, "nature abhors a vacuum". The missing part of the body exists, at the same time, on the "map" that is imprinted within the complex structures of the brain and the mind (Ramachandran, 1998; Melzack, 2006).

This chapter further explores my theory of the psychomatrix and establishes the meaning of the metaphor of the phantom, which is a manifestation of the missing object and an endeavour to make whole the body/self or the mind/self image or map that I will use throughout my theory. In this chapter, I also begin to look at the duality of consciousness, phenomenological and psychological, narcissism, perversion and self-preservation, and the existence of the paradox of pain and pleasure.

My exploration of the neuromatrix in Chapter Two will aid my discussion in this chapter which will be put in relation to my theory of the psychomatrix. The aim will be to examine the phenomenon of pain towards an explanation of the subject-pain (object) relationship.

Chapter Five will discuss the significance of the chronic pain syndrome as found in fibromyalgia. Here I will discuss the conversion between psychological pain and physical pain. I will explore the process of the mind transforming an acute physical trauma into a psychological trauma, (Freud, 1925e; Gamsa, 1994). Physical pain triggers psychological trauma as dose psychological trauma trigger physical ailments that in turn trigger the process of chronic suffering or being in pain. Chronic suffering is the minds repetition of the original trauma—not the actual physical or psychological impact or event, but the reaction of the mind and body matrices—provoking the state of suffering or *being in pain* as opposed to *having pain*. This is by no means an attempt to discount the very reality of chronic pain suffering that some individuals experience as part of having a serious disease such as cancer or rheumatoid arthritis. It can be evidenced in this scenario, the emotional system of the mind striving to gain or regain unity or wholeness, which, again, is impossible thus, resulting in chronic suffering.

Chapter Six will examine addiction, as defined as a set of self-destructive, repetitive, compulsive behaviours. I will discuss two case studies of addiction that will be examined from the perspective of this being another form of neurosis, of a narcissistic occupation that is between the subject and his pain—self-destructive, repetitive, compulsive behaviour—where, again, the object of desire is pain although, an addict will tell you that it is his desire for comfort, pleasure, escape and therefore, management of his pain or suffering. I will explore the subject's desire for control of his internal and external environment, in relation to his pain. Pain, I propose, is the object that is desired by means of the drug as well as other compulsive self-destructive behaviour. I will examine the behaviour of seeking and ingesting. We will also explore the other side of addiction from a perspective of deprivation—a seeking to destroy by starvation with an aim to annihilate the self that is perceived as a "parasite" and a hindrance to gaining pleasure as well as a vehicle of revenge on the object of desire. There is the question of self-preservation—however the more important question is which "self", (Pontalis, 1981) is being preserved, and why? The processes of addictions relegate the pains of real life issues to a shadowy background that becomes a *hum*—that is deafening at times, but managed within the intoxication of indulgence or deprivation—where pain and pleasure lose their boundaries. I will examine the perverse use of the body to be in pain, and the satisfaction of unconscious masochistic desires with the aim to achieve what is beyond pleasure, which is not more pleasure but pain (Freud, 1920g).

My book is not an effort to discuss any particular type of pain or processes of pain, but instead it is to examine the concept of relationship. It is an endeavour to evidence that the subject has a relationship with pain which is pervasive throughout the many levels and dimensions of his identity and existence. My concept of the psychomatrix, derived from Freud's psychosexual theory and Melzack's theory of the neuromatrix, is significant in that it organises the Freudian topographies within the matrix of the unconscious. The methodology, for the most part, is the examination of case studies from a Freudian psychoanalytic model of pain.

CHAPTER ONE

Pain—a vital sign of life?

Introduction

Pain has become such a vital force in the world that it is now considered to be the *fifth vital sign*. Vital signs are an essential part of life. They are the measures of various physiological statistics, often taken by health professionals, in order to assess the most basic body functions. This entails recording the four most essential vital signs: body temperature, pulse rate or heart rate, blood pressure, and respiratory rate.

> To improve pain management the Veterans Health Administration launched the "Pain as the 5th Vital Sign" initiative in 1999, requiring a pain intensity rating (0 to 10) at all clinical encounters. (Mularski et al., 2006, p. 607)

A conference of the *International Association for the Study of Pain* (August/September 2010) presented the conception of a fifth vital sign of life—pain. There are some scientists and healthcare professionals who agree; however, there are those who do not approve of this. In accepting pain as a vital sign of life, is it right or wrong? We do not know. What is relevant is that pain exists in such a way in our world that it cannot be ignored, forgotten, set aside, or escaped. It is part of our minds and our brains and bodies. Just as we breathe, so we feel pain. Nevertheless, is this saying that we *need* pain and that it is essential to our survival, just as we need our breath and blood to flow through us?

It is still early days for this conception and so the *motive* for it has not been established from my perspective. Suffice it to say that this too is, inevitably, another complication added to the psychological reality of our existence and sense of identity. Throughout my book, I propose that pain is an essential part of our existence and our lives: therefore, on the one hand, it is a "vital" sign, however, can it be added to the same categories of blood pressure and respiration or does it need to be assessed as a separate entity? This is yet another debate that has recently taken on a new presence within the scientific community.

A literature search for an historical account of pain has left me with one main conclusion: in order to do this justice the history of pain, rich with all its religious, folkloric, philosophical and scientific data, would have to be set out in many volumes. There has never been a period of time in the history of the world, as we know it, when the topic of pain, particularly chronic pain, has not been a complex and varied entity within people's lives. Pain has always, as far as I can see, occupied the human race due to its elusiveness and mystery, terror, awe and pleasure. It has been relegated to the space of the uncanny and yet it compels an addictive interest.

Historical perspectives on pain

There are, however, a number of authors who have delved into this and compellingly written about the history of the theories and mechanisms of pain. There have been and continue to be various endeavours to bring clarity to the linkage between psychological and physical pain. There are questions about the meaning and the significance of pain within the day to day lives of individuals that have only touched the surface of scientific discoveries. Scientists and researchers such as Melzack and Wall (1965), Melzack (1993, 1996, 2006), Merskey (1965, 1985), Merskey and Spear (1967), Morris (1991), Gamsa (1993), Ramachandran (1994, 1998), Rey (1995), Porter (1997), Liebeskind (1991), Finger and Hustwit (2003), Flor (2009), and numerous others have contributed to the following brief account of my findings.

In ancient times people believed that pain was a mysterious curse related to evil magic. The treatment of which was left to priests and sorcerers who were, nonetheless, well versed in the art of using pressure, heat, water, and sun, to treat pain. Along came the Greek and Roman intellectual input and wisdom that proposed that pain was a sensation, and that the brain and nervous system played a part in producing the perception of pain. Still a new concept, this did not gain much popularity until the Middle Ages. During this period, and the Renaissance, the Western world, particularly Europe, witnessed an increase in the movement of peoples and an increase in population. This brought with it a boom in trading and the sophistication of its courts and the planning of its cities.

There was, however, a down side to all of this mingling and trading—an increase in diseases such as leprosy, the plague and the deterioration in mental health (madness). Scholars and medical intellects of the time categorised these illnesses into four groups: frenzy, mania, melancholy, and fatuity (a lack of intelligence or thought combined with self-satisfaction). The dark and dismal Middle Ages lapsed back to a dependence on ancient folklore and misrepresentations of the remnants of classical learning and knowledge, ignoring the progress of ideologies that had been flowing along through the ages thus far.

Better gains were made in the Renaissance. Intellectuals from this period disapproved of their predecessors, embracing, anew, the lessons and ideologies of classical Greece. They advanced into the new era with an enlightened understanding of how to treat pain and disease. Of the curious intellectuals of the time, Leonardo da Vinci (1452–1519) proposed that the spinal cord was responsible for transmitting sensations to the brain, and the brain in turn was the central organ that was responsible for registering sensations, such as pain.

The seventeenth century experienced further intellectual stimulation and saw a rise in philosophical ideologies. However, this also brought about controversial debates regarding the understanding of the mind/body relationships. For example, Descartes (1596–1650), who in 1664 first described a "pain pathway", was first to identify the "specificity theory" and the idea that pain follows one fixed pathway. Modern research was spring boarded from research such as this, in spite of some misconceptions based on the specificity model. His theory (such as developed by Galileo) was that the body was like a machine that could be studied. Another researcher, Thomas Willis (1621–1675), who has been called the founder of neuroanatomy and neurophysiology, attempted to map mental functions onto particular areas of the brain, laying a foundation for Freud's neurological (and psychological) work in *A Project for a Scientific Psychology* (1950a).

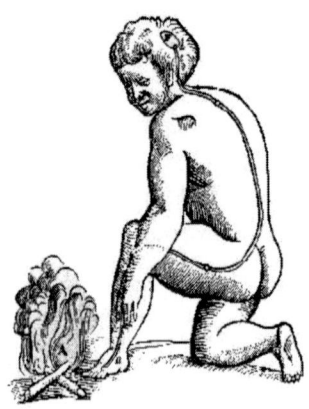

Figure 1. From René Descartes. L'homme de René Descartes. Paris: Charles Angot (1664).

The eighteenth century, known also as the period of "enlightenment", saw many epidemics that raged across Europe resulting in soaring mortality rates. In spite of this, there was an air of heightened hope, as well. This era came to be hailed as the "golden age of quackery" though, as it also witnessed the rise and fall of many medical trends lacking sound and proven theories, such as those of Mesmer (1734–1815) and animal magnetism.

In the nineteenth century, most people expected to experience pain in their lives. They relied on religion, faith, and their own personal resilience to endure their sufferings. Pain was accepted, simply, as a way of life. For example, women endured labour pain and considered it a spiritual experience that would make them better human beings.

As time advanced so did scientific research and discoveries— particularly in pain relief. However, people began to think outside the box of religion, folklore, and faith. They wanted to know what was behind their diseases as well as cures for them. The search for a cure for pain, in the world of science and medicine, opened many doors not least were those into inquiries about the philosophies of life such as, the meaning of life and existence as seen in the rise in popularity of the writings of philosophers such as, Schopenhauer (1788–1860), Kierkegaard (1813–1855) and Nietzsche (1844–1900).

Medical scientists and researchers of the nineteenth century made further advances into pain medication and treatment. Discoveries were made into the pain relieving, benefits of drugs such as opium, morphine, codeine, and cocaine. Felix Hoffmann (1868–1946) was a chemist and one such researcher who developed aspirin (sodium salicylate) which, to this day, is the most commonly used pain reliever. He wished to develop an analgesic, without the side effects of the herbal remedies that were being used, to help his father who suffered with rheumatic pains. I dare say that his father was relieved!

Around this same period, another pain killer was in development and gaining popularity—chloroform (nitrous oxide—laughing gas). This was popular with Queen Victoria during childbirth as she was of the opinion—a wise one at that—that pain during childbirth was not a necessity for the salvation of the soul! Other anaesthetics were developed although there were some physicians who were not completely confident in performing surgery on a comatose patient. There was, in addition, the fear of the potential risk of death from overdose of the anaesthetic.

The twentieth century marched to the tune of further developments in every area of medicine, particularly pain-relieving medicine. The creativity of pharmaceutical companies insured that drugs were starting to be custom-designed to block specific pain mechanisms with fewer side effects. Molecular structures were being manipulated to create and develop drugs for every kind of pain—from neuropathic to psychological pain. By the time the twentieth century was shunted out there were numerous options for pain relief. Pain was no longer a necessity for the salvation of the human soul, and there was no longer the need to endure unnecessary pain. In fact, a pain-free life was the "right" of the human race, and they were going to do whatever it took to be rid of it.

Pain medication, such as aspirin, was widely prescribed. There were other drugs such as aspirin-like, non-steroidal anti-inflammatories (NSAIDs), like ibuprofen and naproxen for mild to moderate pains. Narcotics such as morphine and codeine continue to be prescribed for severe pains.

Considering the vast progress in pharmacological remedies for pain, it is clear to see that by now pain was believed, primarily, to be a physiological and therefore medical, challenge and the responsibility rested with science and the medical world to bring about a pain-free society.

About fifty or so years ago, the specificity theory dominated the study of pain. Dr. Henry Beecher (1904–1976) began an investigation into the validity of this theory and the relationships between subjective psychological states and objective drug responses. Much of his research was done while working with the severely wounded during World War II. When he resumed his work and research after the war, he discovered that significantly fewer soldiers with severe wounds in the combat hospitals complained about intense pain that warranted the administration of morphine, in comparison to the higher number of trauma victims with less severe wounds, who complained about intense pain that warranted the administration of the same drug.

He proposed that the differences in the intensity of pain were not contingent upon the severity of the injury (the sensory stimulus/input) but, instead, had much to do with the *meaning* associated with the injury.

At the time, of course, attacks of the phantom limb pain were common among veterans from the Vietnam war. A significant number of veterans suffered traumatic amputations that caused them continuous experiences of pain in the missing limb.

Advances in pain therapy became the focus of research. In 1965, Melzack and Wall began collating historical data to progress their own extensive scientific research into the multidimensional phenomenon of pain. They proposed that pain was not just something that happened to the body. They soon introduced their "gate control theory" and explained that pain is modulated by past experiences. Once a stimulus has triggered a pain it "opened the pain gate"; however, there were other factors that contributed to the perception of pain. Their work went beyond Descartes' specificity theory to evidence that the brain and the central nervous system played integral and active roles in receiving, modulating, and transmitting pain impulses. Bodily functions for pain were proposed and consequently more advanced pharmacological and surgical interventions were developed for the relief of pain. It was Melzack and Wall's theory that rejuvenated and progressed research from the 1970s onward to the many aspects of pain including physiological, psychological, and emotional.

In the 1990s, Melzack's further research brought him to his discovery of the neuromatrix. He proposed that we all possess an innate "neuromatrix", consisting of a large number of interconnected neurons (as discussed previously). These analyse sensory information in the brain, which in turn provides the perception of sensations—such as pain. The neurosignature is created in the matrix and provides the body/self unity. It tells the brain that the experiences of the sensations are from the "self" and translates the stimuli to be either a threat or a warning. The neurosignature triggers action to maintain the integrity of the body/self unity. Freud's and Melzack and Wall's neurological research urged the consideration of the psychological and emotional dimensions of pain and pain processing.

The twenty-first century heralded in models of cognitive behaviour pain management due to increasing discoveries of the influence of the psychological functions of the mind on the body and the brain. Gamsa (1993) states that:

> [T]he study of pain as a discipline began only in the last half century. As sensory models of pain gave way to multi-dimensional explanations, psychological influences on the perception of pain came to be well accepted. The dominant schools of thought in the discipline of psychology gave impetus to the study of psychological factors in pain. (p. 5)

As we can see, pain has persisted as an integral part of our lives. When Freud began his research and work into the complexities of the human mind his intention was, as it had been of scientists before him, to relieve pain. His effort to invent a drug to relieve pain (Freud's *Cocaine Papers*, 1963), physical and psychological, proved to be unsuccessful. We should be glad for this, as his change of direction into meta-psychology and psychoanalysis proved to be of vital import and continues to contribute to the excavation of new ideas and further comprehension of his original theories and concepts of neurology and psychology.

The main objective of this overview of the process of establishing the vitality of pain through time was to evidence that the focus of any research, for a cause and remedy for pain, has been based on the observable, tangible symptoms. Anything other than obvious was delegated, and still is to some degree, to the uncanny, unexplained and unacceptable.

The question of the importance of pain seems to have travelled a similar path to the ethics and mores of sexuality and how unconscious and conscious thoughts and behaviour impact on our lives and daily functioning as human beings. The build-up and release of energy, I propose, is a key element in pain and is pervasive throughout all dimensions of human sexuality. In fact, pain is at the heart of human sexuality. As such, it has been part and parcel of the controversies which our societies have suffered and debated throughout history.

I propose that as it became more and more evident, somewhere in the course of humanity's history, that pain was a significant aspect of the quality of pleasure; a new paradigm began to be set, which in time dictated that pain needed to be "controlled". Pain, it seems, has become an entity that can be used as a means to a variety of ends—whether political, social, or personal. This is at the heart of my argument. It is the same with drugs. Drugs aid in relieving acute or chronic pain, whether psychological or physical or both, and in many cases also have the side effects of causing a sense of pleasure, hence the need for drugs to be "controlled". Consequently, it so happens that the outcome of controlling pain, as well as controlling drugs has an (incidental) effect of controlling the quantity and quality of pleasure (relief from pain) an individual experiences. The subject's relationship with his pain similarly is one of "control" and "limitations" which acts as a defence against overwhelming issues in his internal as well as external environments. He needs his pain as a baby needs his mother, for comfort and protection. Pain is who he is and this impacts on his existence.

Being in pain versus having pain

More than a hundred years ago, in 1895, when Freud set out to prove his psychological pain theories, he also began from a neurological premise. In *A Project for a Scientific Psychology* (1950a), he began with an attempt to develop a neurological formulation to explain the psychological processing of pain. However, he continued to encounter barriers in his research when trying to identify a (scientific) psychological processing "centre" in the brain. When he finally abandoned the *Project* at the turn of the nineteenth century, he had discovered the phenomenon of the psyche which began a new trend of practice in the medical world. His frustration that he was not able to explain these "pain" affects from a neurological perspective may have been one of the reasons which drove him to psychoanalysis. It appears that he resolved, at the time, that there were some phenomena that could not be explained from a neurological perspective, although the physical and the psychological were somehow interconnected.

Scientists have agreed that an individual's psychological make-up influences how they experience pain—physical pain. It has also been acknowledged that psychological trauma of any kind impacts the emotional system resulting in a variety of mental distress and mental health problems which in turn affect the physical state. Talk therapies may relieve the pressures of unexpressed trauma and medication may be administered to decrease physiological symptoms to bring about temporary psychological relief. However, as Freud discovered, emotional pain, caused by psychological or physical trauma, remains a part of the individual's make-up, bleeding through into their thoughts and behaviour, pervasive throughout all dimensions of daily functioning.

Upon examining Melzack's concept of the neuromatrix as well as Freud's neurological concepts in his *Project*, what I generally saw was the similarity in the explanations of the neurological systems of processing. What I also identified is that Freud's concept of the mind and its topographies was an attempt to map emotional and psychological pain processes that could not be explained neurologically. One of the main aspects of the neuromatrix is the mapping of the body/self whole across the structure of the brain. It is also an explanation of how the neurological systems work to keep this body/self map/imprint intact in the brain. If a part of the body is missing as for example, in the case of amputation, the system reacts in such a way so as to maintain the "whole" map or imprint in the brain. The results of this, is a painful affect at the sight of the missing limb. The effort of the brain in this quest maintains not only physical pain or painful experiences, but also psychological distress, long after the actual trauma and physical healing (Ramachandran, 1998). The pain of this experience has become part of the emotional system causing distress, as it is unable to be resolved. The only option is to learn to manage this pain and function in spite of this.

According to Melzack (1993), the mapping system in the brain represents an image of the body. In other words, this is what the body ought to look like and where every aspect of the body should be situated; so, for example, if I need to lift something my brain will identify on its whole body/self map where the lifting capabilities are assumed to be found (arms, hands, fingers muscles, etc.) and send a message to lift. I think that this brain map may be situated in the *imaginary realm* (Lacan, 1977; Evans, 2006) as in the mirror stage where "the baby sees its own image as whole". However, the baby struggles with the contrast between what he sees in the specular (whole and independent) image and his *un*coordination (and dependence), which he experiences "as a fragmented body". This experienced discrepancy creates a threat of "fragmentation" to his ego, the sense of a whole self (Evans, 2006, p. 115).

The discrepancy between what exists in the brain's mapping system and the body with the missing limb creates a similar threat to the body self/ego. I propose that the unconscious desire to maintain the real is expressed in the pain experienced in the phantom limb. The phantom limb, in other words becomes a metaphor or symbol of the desire for the whole, which is the real of the map within the brain as well as the unconscious. Therefore, the real can only be expressed in the (symbolic) language of pain, as it is unknowable.

The loss of a limb is not (willingly) accepted by the brain as it struggles to maintain the whole self. Therefore, even though the "map" indicates that the *road* exists, the real fact is that the *road* no longer (or never did) exists. The brain and the mind struggle to maintain its *map* and the *reality* of an intact body/self and ignore the loss—which in turn is, as has been evidenced, a painful process. We are so influenced by what is acceptable or reality within social constructs that the loss of a limb is (emotionally and psychologically) unacceptable. It is also a *painful* reminder of the "original" loss and desire that lies within the unconscious.

My argument, after also examining Freud's theory of the mind, its topographies and influence on cognitive processing and behaviour (actions/reactions), is that there may exist, similar to the neuromatrix, a *psychomatrix*. This would be the matrix within which the psyche functions to maintain a certain emotional balance (or "whole"), allowing one to function. However, since we know that according to psychoanalytic theory it is impossible to reach this "whole" or ultimate balance or ultimate pleasure, the individual continues to experience a certain level of "emotional pain" throughout his life. And further, I believe that it is possible that the *psychomatrix* functions, mainly, in the service of the psyche and works toward managing emotional pain. In connection with this, my main argument is that it is not the actual pain sensation, whatever the cause; it is the individual's *relationship* to the pain that is the primary element influencing his behaviour.

In cases where there is the condition that prevents an individual from experiencing physical pain (i.e., congenital insensitivity to pain (CIP), McMurray, 1975) the effect is of distress and a painful emotional state that physical pain is not felt. This is still pain felt even though it is psychological pain experienced within the desire to *have pain* in order to make sense of the physical and to understand the *being in pain*.

The similarities in the theories of Melzack and Freud, over a century apart, prompted me to propose that in creating his theory of the topography of ego, id, and superego within the unconscious, Freud set out a framework for a matrix. Within this matrix are the innate "instincts" of the life and death drives which are akin to signatures or patterns of psychological and emotional processing which cannot be re-created. However, in order to allow for the *psychosignatures* to be modulated to, in turn, facilitate learning and development/growth, the ego, id, and superego, mechanisms within the matrix, act in the capacity of facilitators allowing this modulation. The input of information from experiences, from birth (perhaps even from conception) onwards, and output of thoughts and behaviours—actions and reactions/responses—are thus influenced. Freud created the topographies to facilitate an understanding of the psychological system and that of emotions—namely pain which is the result of "loss of the object". This pain appears to be akin to pain that results from a physical injury; in fact the reactions and affects are the same. As has been evidenced in further research (i.e., Gamsa, 1994), physical and psychological functioning is correlative. For example, as evidenced in Freud's theory of hysteria, a physical symptom is the manifestation of an (unresolved, unconscious) emotional trauma.

This is significant to my book, not because there is one type of pain or the other (physical or psychological) but instead, that both types of pain "register" in the psychological system and become part of the emotional make-up and in turn, influences how we respond to stimuli, whether it is physical or psychological. My argument therefore, is that the initial response to pain registers, primarily from an emotional premise, which is the relational sphere of being human.

In his *Project* (1950a) Freud discussed the impact of and the responses to internal and external stimuli, through the nervous system. He postulated that responses to stimuli are facilitated by permeable and impermeable neurons. This process creates the environment that allows for the formation of memory, perception, and motives thereof, for example, facilitating the satisfaction of the "exigencies of life" such as hunger (p. 297). Satisfaction of hunger would be one of the innate drives, which are part of the creation of the psychosignature, and would work toward this end. In the case of hunger not readily being satisfied, the "pain" of anxiety is clear in the cries of a hungry baby.

Freud (1950a) proposed, initially, that pain was a failure of the "contrivances" of the "biological nature that have limits to their efficiency" (p. 306). Therefore, it was the failure of the physical body's protective mechanisms that caused pain. However, what of psychological pain? He wanted to understand the pain that was obvious in the occurrence of anxiety.

In the case of an anxiety pain response there was no physical "peripheral stimulation", however, Freud posited that perhaps there is a similarity in that:

> the intense cathexis of longing which is concentrated on the missed object (a cathexis which steadily mounts up because it cannot be appeased) creates the same economic conditions as are created by an injured part of the body. Thus, the fact of the peripheral causation of physical pain can be left out of the account. (ibid., p. 171)

Pain, therefore, has its roots in (innate as well as learned) physical as well as psychological experiences. Therefore, when we speak of psychological and/or emotional pain, the answer goes beyond the awareness of a sudden or an acute event that causes psychological or physical impact. The definition of pain, as discussed in my book, is that it is a *conglomerate* of past, traumatic, neurobiological, psychological, and emotional imprints that influence our day to day life—pain as in *suffering* or *being in pain.*

From these formulations, I propose that there is a distinct possibility for the existence of what I have named a *psychomatrix* within the structure of the (unconscious) mind. I conceptualise it as being patterns of pain (loss—abandonment, grief, rejection, desire) imprinted in infancy which form their own psychological and emotional "neural loops". As pain is triggered these "loops" become more ingrained, as memory triggers are translated and coded to create a continuous experience of *suffering* and *being in pain* on the map of our emotional self within the unconscious mind. This is also true for positive emotions, such as love and joy, however I argue that pain is the primary, and most significant, emotion that needs to be understood in order to understand the others that are triggered on the same neural—psychological and physical—pathways.

This is based on the concept of Melzack's neuromatrix which is within the structure of the brain. I propose that regardless of how one experiences pain the experience is imprinted in the emotional system in the unconscious mind, and what I propose is a matrix within which the *psychomatrix* resides. Within the psychomatrix is formed the *psycho-signature,* which figures into the processing of the conglomerate of pain. As the mind attempts to resolve certain traumas (depending on what is triggered during the course of life), the emotional state is activated by the activities within the psychomatrix. Since it is not possible to fully resolve the trauma (to go back to the point before it took place), the pain continues, as emotional residues or imprints are left behind—creating a sense of *suffering* or *being in pain.* This brings me to my main argument, which is that it is not this feeling or sensation of pain as such, but the *relationship*—the complexities of the awareness of this presence—to this pain that impacts the individual's sense of existence, as well as his sense of identity.

Freud's *Project* has been reviewed and further investigated by several researchers, such as Pontalis (1981) and Solms (1998) and appreciated for its neurological as well as psychological contributions to modern day theoretical formulation. He laid the foundation for research which has taken us into a better understanding of the psychological and emotional mechanisms of human development within which rests the primary aspects of identity and existence. The correlations to neurology are significant and would not be understood without the "science" of psychology and Freud's efforts to marry the two.

In exploring Freud's work, Pontalis (1981) identified that there were three phases that the psychoanalytic explanation of pain traversed. He acknowledged Freud's formulation of object loss being the prevalent category and in the first phase, anxiety and pain have both been identified in relation to object loss. However, in the second phase he lists four categories in relation to pain: 1) Freud's *Project* identified pain as the consequence of a breach in the protective shield; 2) pain acts as a "constant instinctual excitation"; 3) pain is independent of the experience of need; and 4) pain emanates from the "periphery". At this point, Freud did not connect pain to the anxiety reaction in object loss. In the third phase, however, he states that Freud's further research brought him to a new understanding of pain. Here, Freud saw that the expenditure of energy would be the same "whether in the case of cathexis of longing concentrated upon the missing or lost object or in the case of cathexis concentrated upon an injured part of the body" (1950a, pp. 197–198).

The significance of this explanation to my proposal is that even in 1895 Freud identified that the effect of pain was the same whether it was physical or psychological.

Freud's scientific research, in the late nineteenth and early twentieth centuries, as well as that of other scientists such as Melzack and Wall (1965, 1996), Melzack (1993, 2001), Livingston (1976), Merskey (1965, 1985) Merskey and Spear (1967), Pontalis (1981), Gamsa (1994), Solms (1998), Pribram and Gill (1976, 1998) Ramachandran (1998), Schore (2001), and others, has shown that the mechanisms of the body and the brain are influenced by biologically embedded coding, and the endogenous development of processing mechanisms. Melzack and Wall (1965) acknowledge the significance of Freud's point of view even though their research is neuroscientific. To validate their scientific view they acknowledge that "even Freud regarded pain with a major psychological basis as also having an organic substrate such as muscle tension" (p. 31). The perspective that pain has to have a neuro-biological component continues to be a paradigm that urges researchers to provide evidence for even those psychological phenomena that are unexplainable. The definition of psychological and emotional pain thus, remains elusive even in this century although, one sees *suffering* or *being in pain* everywhere and as Freud did in his clinical work, we continue to see our patients' emotional suffering as something which needs to be investigated from an emotional/psychological perspective.

I will explore these theories to map the excitatory and inhibitory processes of pain, including Melzack's theory of the existence of a "neuromatrix" in relation to physical and psychological pain processes and perception. Melzack explains that the brain perceives the body as a certain "whole". Even when there is a "cut" or dismemberment, either from birth or caused during one's life, the brain's mechanism continues to perceive the body as a "whole", therefore behaving as if it is a "whole" (1993, p. 621). This phenomenon, I believe, is what figures into the notion of "mourning a loss", and the efforts of the neurological and psychological systems to compensate for what was once perceived as an attached, essential member of a dynamic subject—the body and the mind. Melzack (1993) stated that "[t]he brain does more than detect and analyse inputs; it generates perceptual experience even when no external inputs occur" (ibid., p. 628).

This compares to what Pontalis (1981) identified as the "third phase" of Freud's theory of pain, as stated above. I argue that these "perceptual experiences", although detected in the mechanisms of physiology, become part of the emotional and psychological dynamics of the development of the subject's relationship with pain, where they are further translated in the identification of self and the meaning of existence.

Scientific research since Freud has progressed to explain the many, if not all the mysteries of pain, particularly of the relationship between physical and psychological pain. Further research continues into the complexities of emotions and feelings within the cognitive mechanisms involving pain. Since the beginning of their work in the 1960s, Melzack and Wall have introduced "the gate control theory of pain", theories on the "phantom limb syndrome" and the "neuromatrix" (Melzack, 1965–1993).

Freud's effort to create a framework to explain psychology from a scientific point of view and to impress the correlations and influence of neurobiology on psychology in his *Project* has not, after all, been in vain, as his theory is articulated by ongoing research. An example of this is found in Pribram's writing suggesting that:

> Freud emphasized not the drive basis of motivation, but its basis in the memory-motive structure developed in the core brain (the basal forebrain), *not* the cortex. Only later, when Freud began to believe that memory became distorted by the surge of hormones at puberty, did he ascribe an overwhelming importance to drives (by that time called the id …). […] Clark Hull took up Freud's later emphasis on drive and applied it to learning. (1998, p. 13)

In examining Freud's 1895 *A Project for a Scientific Psychology* (1950a), Schore (2001) stated that Freud's germinal hypothesis concerning the regulatory structures and dynamics of the system unconscious has translated its significance to the theory of attachment. Here is one primary example where the pain of *object loss* becomes visible and begins to enter the dimension of relationships which is the core element in the processes of life, particularly in the management of trauma—*suffering/ being in pain*.

This will set the stage for further discussions in subsequent chapters, and the exploration of Freud's theories of the unconscious and sexuality, which impact on every aspect of human behaviour. Throughout his works—from his all-important *A Project for a Scientific Psychology* (1950a), *The Interpretation of Dreams* (1900a), *Three Essays on the Theory of Sexuality* (1905d), *On Narcissism: an Introduction* (1914c), *Beyond the Pleasure Principle* (1920g), *The Ego and the Id* (1923b) to *Inhibitions, Symptoms and Anxiety* (1926d) and *Civilization and its Discontents* (1930a)—Freud outlined the significance of the formation of relationships throughout the stages of an individual's development and its central role in human sexuality and the unconscious.

The relationship between sexuality and the unconscious is an essential component in analysing the subject's relationship with his pain. Pain becomes an entity in the subject's life, from the first moment of the experience of loss, which evolves through the developmental stages. It is an object of attention which is brought by the subject into every life event and circumstance. It is an object such as a "partner"—one who compels pleasure—and demands the same emotional attention. It is thus a key element in the subject's unconscious and sexuality as any other relational entity in the subject's life. Therefore, pain has the power to inspire or destroy. Freud has evidenced throughout his work that we are lived by our unconscious and its drives in the sense that they determine all human activities and the trajectory of each individual's course of life.

Relationships seem to be the source of one's major traumatic experiences and the basis of one's psychological pain. If we see ourselves in relation to others the question is: what do we see? As a sexual being the primary view the subject has of himself, then, is sexual. As relational beings, we locate ourselves and the purpose of our existence through our connections and interactions with others. Due to this, fear of loss (and actual loss) figures as the central point of one's pain. I propose that as one develops these relationships to others, one develops a relationship with pain.

The dichotomy of pleasure and pain and the impossibility of satisfaction in pleasure will be evidenced in my discussions on Freud's theories on loss, perversion, and narcissism as well as his theory on the life and death instincts. The discussion will inform my argument of the existence of a psychomatrix and its significance and influence on the subject-pain relationship and behaviour. As the neuromatrix embodies the working of the body/self, the psychomatrix, specifically, embodies the workings of the mind/self and the conglomerate of pain. In examining the subject-pain relationship, it would then follow that I also acknowledge the notion of pain as the object (of desire). Since this notion and the significance of the objectification of pain, is what gives my book its premise, this thread will run through my whole investigation.

The word "relationship", by and large, has an emotional association within the varied, be it positive or negative, scenarios of human interactions, between the subject and his significant object or objects of attention. For example, one's parent, child, sexual partner, and so on. There are also those objects of wider relationships within society such as religious faiths and cultural beliefs in gods and devils—higher entities that give one a sense of boundaries, accountability, protection, security, escape as well as a sense of euphoria or despair—and other powers that influence one's life. All of these, I propose, invariably affect one's more personal relationships but especially the relationship with one's pain and therefore one's "self", and the meaning of one's existence.

The relationship between an individual and pain, then, is no different as it entails all the emotional dimensions of any other relationship including the sense of responsibility—herein lies the meaning of *being in pain*. Pain is what influences all aspects of our lives—our thoughts and behaviour. However, the decision to act in spite of (or because of or due to) our pain, is a responsibility that lies within the individual's sphere of control. Therefore, working through certain past, unresolved emotional trauma can be beneficial in gaining a better comprehension of why *suffering/being in pain* is part of our lives and the processes of our thoughts and behaviour.

Psychoanalytic and psychological research has made great progress in the study of the self, neurosis, and psychosis, the unconscious, repression, anxieties, and defence mechanisms, human sexuality, relationships, and the duality of pain and pleasure. However, it has yet to take a firm stand on the subject of psychological and emotional pain. When we treat someone for depression or anxieties or even, addiction, chronic pain, and phantom limb syndromes, we fail to speak in terms of the individual *being in pain*. It is usually about *having pain* as in *having a disease*.

A disease model is a model of chronic, enduring, persistent problems that need to be treated on a continuum of pathology—a process and progression of a condition that is separate and a deviation from *the normal*.

The label itself may lead to significant emotional trauma and distress. The ramifications are serious and may affect certain lifestyle decisions, for example, decisions around having children, career choice, and attitude toward oneself and others. The benefit of diagnosing someone as diseased would be in linking certain symptoms to a legitimate disease and clarification of personal responsibility, and improved access to appropriate health care (Temple, McLeod, Gallinger, & Wright, 2001, p. 807).

To say that an individual has a disease due to his being in psychological and emotional pain would be to condemn him to a lifetime without hope, throwing him into a situation that compels him to make decisions that are psychologically or physically unbeneficial to living a productive life. I would argue that it is essential to realise that this pain will impact on all dimensions of one's life. For example, a recent study indicates that psychological distress impacts on long-term disability consistently and that "depression and stress individually were both partial mediators in the pain-disability relationship" (Hall et al., 2011, p. 1049).

It needs to be emphasised that, even though the scenarios I discuss in this book are those that could be said to be of individuals with diseases, I do not consider their respective psychological and emotional pain to be a disease. Rather, it is to demonstrate that psychological and emotional pain (even though these may be caused by physical, psychological and or environmental trauma) can become viewed as an attribute of one's life from a perspective of it being a disease that, in turn, may have a detrimental effect on a person's identity and how he views himself. I do not intend to depict *pain*, which I discuss in this book to be pathological and outside the "normal" sphere of human existence. On the contrary, in reference to Schopenhauer's (1969) theory on pain, it is a necessary component of our existence that is always with us, and needs to be understood to inspire and enrich life (pp. 318–319). I propose that we cannot hope to "understand and be inspired" by something unless we have a relationship or emotional connection with it.

Conclusion

My curiosity is sparked by the many patients, clients, and others who live rewarding and successful lives, in spite of pain (physical and or psychological/emotional). What is the difference between this group of people and those who cannot live with their pain and whose lives are destroyed with a sort of emotional paralysis of the mind? I can, at the same time, appreciate the fact that there are a plethora of cultural, religious, environmental, social, psychological, biological, organic, developmental, and historical factors influencing how one relates to, and thinks and feels about, his own pain. The point to stress is this—*one relates to, thinks and feels*, a certain way about one's own pain. In other words the psychological and emotional make-up of the body, brain, and mind of the individual need to be considered as a whole when considering a treatment process for an individual with a presenting problem of pain—be it a broken bone, a broken heart, a phantom limb, chronic pain, or even an addiction. I view this as significant in understanding that its *affect* (emotional) not *sensation* (physical) is the more important and which figures in the subject-pain connection or *relationship*.

From the beginning of our existence, our unconscious has been storing imprints of memories from our experiences. Into the unconscious, as Freud postulated, are repressed, unacceptable memories—urges and instincts, traumatic events and experiences—a conglomerate which I have named *pain*. Pain, as such, impacts on one as unpleasure or suffering, not one particular experience at a time but as a conglomerate. This overshadows and influences the subject's development, manifesting in its various forms, and levels of painful intensities, as the subject strives to achieve the opposite—pleasure. However, the pain persists in one's life. As Schopenhauer (1969) postulated that at the end of the day the pleasure that is achieved is merely a "deliverance from a pain and so the desire and therefore the pleasure ceases" (p. 319).

The duality of pain and pleasure tend to rule one's progress through life. What is repressed, as Freud (1920g) postulated, in the unconscious, struggles to the surface of consciousness only to be censored by the *reality principle* on its way towards some form of discharge, the aim being pleasure, governed by the *pleasure principle* and what is *beyond the pleasure principle*.

CHAPTER TWO

From Freud's project to Melzack's neuromatrix

Introduction

In this chapter, I shall examine Freud's 1895 *Project* as well as Melzack and Wall's research that began in the 1960s through to Melzack's (1993, 2006) continuing research on pain processing focusing on his theory of the neuromatrix. There will also be references to other researchers such as Pontalis (1981), Pribram and Gill (1976), Solms (1998), Ramachandran (1998), and Schore (2001) to evidence my theory.

The significance in doing so is to examine how the processing of pain, within Freud's theory of his 1895 *Project* and Melzack's theory of the neuromatrix in the 1990s, influences my concept of the existence of the psychomatrix which figures in the subject's relationship with his pain. Here we will also see links between psychological and emotional pain and its development by looking at the activities of the nervous system.

Tracing the similarities between Freud's work in the *Project* and Melzack's concept of the neuromatrix will be an endeavour to identify two issues: (1) that what Freud started to speak about and set down in his work of 1895 laid the scientific foundations for the discoveries that have been made today regarding the links between psychological and neurological pain; and (2) that there are some phenomena within psychic pain that cannot be explained neuro-scientifically. These can only be identified by the manifestations of human behaviour which is, I propose, contingent upon the relationship that the subject develops with his pain.

I argue that *suffering* or *being in pain* betrays the subject-pain relationship which is an entity that exists due to the existence of memory, motive, consciousness and perception. Freud's explanations, in the end, were psychological or rather meta-psychological as he developed psychoanalysis as a treatment for human suffering. As Pribram and Gill (1976) state:

> Clinical theory, better labelled "psychology" (though Freud originally used the term psychology for what is now called metapsychology), encompasses those formulations derived from observations in the analytic situation and stated in the intentional language of motivations and meanings; while metapsychology describes the mechanisms of such mental functioning. (p. 10)

Pain, particularly emotional pain, is an entity that has eluded definition throughout human history. Each age, from antiquity to our modern technological era has had, and has, its own perspective and definition of pain. Be that as it may, pain, it is agreed, is a personal experience and each individual has his own way of contending with it. I propose that the common denominator is that pain is made up of a conglomerate of each individual's experiences, physical or psychological. This pain (subjective though it may be) becomes an entity or object akin to a life partner to be contended with throughout each individual's life. According to Freud's clinical observations, his patients presented with emotional pain due to historical, unresolved, emotional trauma. Their pain took on a variety of forms such as hysterical symptom where, for example, a part of the body functioning would be affected.

As far back in history as the period of the Greek tragedies, as aptly described by Rey (1995), this pain is perceived almost as an independent being which takes possession of the subject, invades it and takes over. Words such as "consuming" and "devouring" were used to qualify the impact of pain on its victim (p. 15).

This period in Greek history is interesting in its depiction and dramatisation of tragedy, pain, and suffering, as pain is viewed as an awesome power. It invokes fear as well as excitement. Pain is likened to a wild, ravaging animal: "it is not possible to tame savage pain because of its intensity and also because one cannot predict when and how it will occur" (ibid., p. 15). The sufferer is the "hunted" and the traditional relationship between man and beast is reversed. Rey explains, "pain stalks its prey and overcomes it at the most convenient moment." Its mission is to kill but before that to make its victim suffer. In the Tragedies pain is an essential dimension that tells of the power of the "will of the gods", leaving the sufferer with no control, but to embrace his suffering, so much so that when the pain is at its worst the sufferer becomes the pain that invades him—he becomes lost and "like a diseased animal on the prowl". He attacks with unrelenting cries—his body writhing and contorting ... "To explain the terrible nature of pain, Greek texts simply say that it is unapproachable." (ibid, p. 15).

Even in present day conception of pain, any pain is looked upon as an outside entity, an object of power to be reckoned with. The relationship may be one of slave and master—subject and object of fear as well as desire—as if the suffering must be just right in order to appease the gods perhaps for greater gains of pleasure. However, we know, from a psychoanalytic point of view, this is not possible. There are no ultimate pleasures but only more pain.

Freud (1905d, 1909d, 1923b, etc.) uses the Greek myth of Oedipus (Sophocles, fifth century BC) as the perfect metaphor to his explanation of psychological and emotional pain. He evidences here his theory of the unconscious and sexuality. He establishes that pain is a component of human development from the beginning of one's life, from birth and the loss of the womb, to death and loss of his life and a return to ultimate equilibrium—to that from which he came. Oedipus is the paradigm for the greatest of human pains, namely the complexities of human relationships. Here there is fear and anxiety, abandonment, loss and depression, love and hate, jealously, rage, guilt, and punishment. Oedipus seems to have traversed his whole life with nothing less than this *conglomerate* of pain.

What is it that compels one to choose a certain path in life? The answer is an insurmountable task. However, one thing that Freud seemed to be sure of and evidenced in his work is that whatever is imprinted in the unconscious impacts our decisions and behaviour. The unconscious mind is the driving force in one's life. Within it lies the conglomerate of experiences which make up the entity of emotional pain. I argue that, hence this is what the subject develops a relationship with. This is what impacts on the process of his psychological and more essentially his emotional development.

Freud's project for a scientific psychology

In *A Project for a Scientific Psychology* (1950a), Freud proposed that the cognitive mechanisms of normal and abnormal mental phenomena could be explained through an orderly and rigorous study of brain systems. He pursued a scientific explanation for causes of human behavioural manifestations that were observed in his clinical work. He set out to explain his scientific theory in his 1895 *Project* and stated that "[t]he intention is to furnish a psychology that shall be a natural science: that is, to represent psychical processes as quantitatively determinate states of specifiable material particles, thus making those processes perspicuous and free from contradiction" (p. 295).

According to Solms (1998), one of the academic problems that Freud faced in those days was that of consciousness and memory. He quotes from Freud's (1891b) monograph on aphasia:

> What then is the physiological correlate of the simple idea emerging or re-emerging? Obviously, nothing static, but something in the nature of a process. This process is not incompatible with localization. It starts at a specific point in the cortex and from there it spreads over the whole cortex along certain pathways. When this event has taken place it leaves behind the possibility of a memory, in the part of the cortex affected. It is very doubtful whether this physiological event is in any way associated with something psychic. Our consciousness contains nothing that would, from the psychological point of view, justify the term "latent memory image." Yet whenever the same cortical state is elicited again, the previous psychic event re-emerges as a memory (p. 4). Freud assumed that the "underlying modifications" must be physical as he "could not conceive of the possibility that something non-conscious could be described as a 'memory'."
>
> It did not make sense to him, at the time, to consider the underlying "modifications" had a psychological basis. Therefore in his *Project* he "… laid the stress in psychology on the somatic processes" (ibid).

However, another major issue was that, at the time, there was a lack of scientific knowledge available linking the somatic to the psychic leaving much to "speculation, imaginings, transpositions, and guesses ..." (ibid., pp. 4–5).

When Freud made the transition from neuropsychology to psychoanalysis he had established in his mind that there were mental processes that could not be explained within the models of physiological processes yet, he hoped that one day there would be. He resigned to making use of what he knew first hand in his clinical observations: "transforming his clinical knowledge into a hypothetical neurological machine, Freud laid the foundation for a future neuropsychology, but the knowledge itself remained psychological" (ibid., p. 8). His key perspective was that there were physical processes as well as psychological processes, some of which were conscious and some were unconscious and the unconscious processes could be inferred by the conscious ones. Consciousness had two features, an external perception of the world and an internal perception of the inner workings of the mind, "which represents the unconscious reality that lies within us in the form of subjective states of awareness—such as memories, beliefs, and desires" (ibid). (Solms, 1998)

In his *Project*, Freud explains that the nervous system relies on the principle of inertia as well as on the "quantity-screens" set up by the "nerve-endings" to filter the impact of stimuli of the external world. "All contrivances of a biological nature have limits to their efficiency, beyond which they fail. This failure is manifested in phenomena which border on the pathological" (p. 306). Thus, he describes the cause of pain neurologically—"a *failure* of the system to protect the subject from the impact of external stimuli". Pain that remains with the subject, beyond the initial impact of a stimulus, is an imprint of the experience left on the memory system of the brain and the mind influencing the judgment process and motivation toward the satisfaction of desire.

Pribram and Gill (1976) have explained that according to the *Project* there are two types of neurons that carry stimuli—permeable and impermeable. The permeable (φ) neurones allow stimuli to pass through and remain unaltered and "by virtue of contact with the environment are primarily responsible for reception and motor discharge" whereas the impermeable (ψ) neurones resist and retain affect, and are "systems in contact with endogenous excitation which are for the most part given over to retention". Freud was most concerned with the impermeable system of neurons because "this selective facilitation is the basis of memory trace". They express Freud's views that:

> [a] psychological theory deserving any consideration must furnish an explanation of "memory". This was described by Freud in neurological terms that all psychological retentions depend on the communication between the impermeable systems of neuronal "contact barriers". (pp. 66–69)

Pribram and Gill (1976) further discuss here that "repeated transmission lowers synaptic resistance" to allow an increase in response to stimuli. However, there is also an increase in what is retained in the nervous system. This was significant in explaining certain psychological activities, such as, memory which is:

> evidently one of the powers which determine and direct its pathway, and, if facilitation were everywhere equal, it would not be possible to see why one pathway should be preferred. We can, therefore, say still more correctly that memory is represented by the differences in the facilitations between the impermeable neurons. (ibid., pp. 66–69)

Memory and motive are then accordingly derived from the impact of internal and external stimuli and the responses of the physiological nervous system. Pribram and Gill (1976) cite Glover (1947) who proposes "that the basic structural concept of psychoanalysis is a memory trace." And that:

> memories are the retrospective aspects of the facilitations; motives the prospective aspects (see Pribram, 1962). In retrospect, facilitations result from and thus reflect the experiences of the organism; prospectively they are feed forward programmes that run themselves off to completion thus guiding motivating behaviour. We must recall in this respect that the Project was written at a time when Freud still believed that the verbal reports of his patients

reflected accurately the actual occurrences they had experienced in childhood. (p. 70–71)

Freud later modified this theory when his findings indicated the perception of his patients' experiences can be "distorted" during the stage of puberty and the development of the drive system.

> These modifications took the form, foreshadowed in the *Project* (p. 316), of an increased abstraction and autonomy of that part of ψ—the "nuclear neurons", the "nucleus of the ψ", a "sympathetic ganglion"—which receives, in the main, the excitations of endogenous origin—the part which is in later writings to becomes the id. (ibid.)

Freud explained that:

> consciousness is the subjective side of one part of the physical processes in the nervous system, namely of the ω [ω = system of perceptual neurons] processes; and the omission of consciousness does not leave psychical events unaltered but involves the omission of the contribution from ω. (p. 311)

The primary processes, the rapid discharge and flow of energy, can be evidenced within mechanisms "such as drive, pain, unpleasure, and the initial production of affect and wish". The secondary processes are "behaviour processes, from wishes which are simple memory-motive structures through the operation of defences and satisfaction, to behaviour controlled by an executive ego" is the accumulation of or "bound" energy caused by "barriers" or "resistance" to discharge. This, in turn, results in the slower discharge of energy. This bound energy, then, is the cathexis that consciousness attaches itself to (ibid., p. 28).

The "nature of the ego" is the complex of neurons, the nuclear neurons that receive endogenous stimuli and regulate these barriers to satisfaction of wishes. The id is part of the make-up of the nucleus of the permeable neuron that receives the stimuli of the "endogenous origin"—the rapid discharge of energy without resistance. The permeable neurons are subdivided to primarily allow perception of the quality of external stimuli, that is colour, texture, shape, taste, and sound. The other reason is to allow for cathexis—the conduction and "periodicity" of the quantity of energy—between the permeable (φ) and impermeable (ψ) neurons.

The "motive structure" depends on the selectivity of contact barriers and affects the "organism's behaviour". Memory is influenced by both endogenous and exogenous stimuli which, in turn, "contribute to the formation of each facilitation". When presented with the "exigencies of life" such as hunger, respiration, and sexuality, from the endogenous stimuli, the "principle of inertia is breached" and must be satisfied by the "external world"—for example, nutrition. The linkage of motive and memory in the structure of the wish is one of the fundamental contributions of psychoanalysis and is significant to the particular conditions that are called "specific actions" that are triggered by an "endogenous stimuli" such as hunger (ibid., pp. 71–89).

Freud's 1895 attempt at mapping out the structures of the nervous system which in turn impacted on the structures of the mechanisms of the psychological system was significant to the identification of the development of patterns of neuron behaviour within the organism. This in turn identified patterns of pathological developments due to excessive stimulus and breaches, or a "breakthrough" in the fidelity of the protective mechanisms causing acute or chronic trauma such as physical/psychological pain or unpleasure.

Freud's work on the *Project* influenced all his subsequent work. His theory of pain is evidenced throughout his work and according to Pontalis (1981):

> one cannot but be aware of the fact that a whole dimension, always present on the horizon of human experience—pain—returns time and again in the work of Freud, almost in spite of himself. The key-text here is certainly *Beyond the Pleasure Principle* (1920g). So what is this remainder, so honestly and imperatively sought by Freud, this something that in the end neither the pleasure principle nor even masochism can quite encompass? What is it that is in the proper sense, beyond the principle of unpleasure-pleasure, if it is not pain? (p. 197)

The pleasure principle is guided by the "principle of constancy" or keeping the "excitation" in the "mental apparatus" down to as low a level as possible. The aim is to avoid unpleasure or stimulation over a certain limit (Freud, 1920g, p. 9). Freud also spoke of the "nirvana principle" that is compelled by the death instinct which is the desire of the organism to return to an inanimate state. Once excitation is satisfied, however, there is a need or desire for further satisfaction as stimuli from life's demands, from within and without the organism, exercise their various pressures. "The nirvana principle", he maintains, is to be attributed to the "death instinct", and its modification into the pleasure principle is due to the influence of the "life instinct" or "libido" (pp. 50–56).

A recent study published by the International Association for the Study of Pain suggests that the *Project* contains "surprisingly precise concepts of the possibility for memory to be represented by long-lasting alterations of synaptic transmission".

It further affirms Freud's *Project* theories by stating that:

> the employment of mathematical models, computer simulations, and experiments on single cerebral neurons have for some time now confirmed Freud's insight, indicating in fact how information is better stored and retained when there is a mere variable degree of synaptic facilitation induced among the thousands of synapses existing in a given neuronal network. (Centonze et al., 2004, p. 311)

Melzack and Wall's neurological theory of pain

The theory of pain has been explored from a variety of perspectives—philosophical, sociological, psychological, and scientific—throughout time, a challenging task that has, even today, been without specific, satisfactory results. However, research continues. Melzack and Wall (1996, pp. 44–46) have identified three possible theories, the first being that "pain is a sensory experience evoked by stimuli" where there is "real or threatened tissue damage". However, this definition falls short because there can be pain whether or not these conditions are present. The second theory "refers to a personal, private sensation of hurt". This, too, was unacceptable as it begs the question, what is "hurt"? The answer would be "pain" and a circular argument ensues. The third seems to be closest to a further understanding of this pervasive entity, and the most significant to this investigation. These two scientists refer to the definition by Merskey (1986), who states that "pain is an unpleasant sensory and emotional dimension of experience associated with actual or potential tissue damage", and appreciates the fact that it mentions the "link between injury and pain", and acknowledges the emotional and sensory dimensions of the experience of pain.

To Melzack and Wall, in 1996, the problem was the usage of the expression "unpleasant", as to them "unpleasant" did not begin to express the reality of the multiple dimensions of this experience that is called "pain". It can make some people scream and fight, undergo crippling, disfiguring operations, or even commit suicide. "What are missing in the word 'unpleasant' are the misery, anguish, desperation, and urgency that are part of some pain experiences. The qualities of 'unpleasantness' are complex and comprise multiple dimensions that have yet to be determined" (1996, p. 45).

One of these dimensions is that of emotional pain that lives in a realm of the psychological systems that influence thoughts and behaviours.

Their summary of these definitions is that the word "pain" represents a *category* of experiences, signifying a multitude of different, unique experiences having different causes, and characterised by different qualities varying along a number of sensory, affective and evaluative dimensions (ibid., p. 46). This work represents a part of the modern day research that has uncovered some essential aspects of the integration of physical and psychological mechanisms, particularly in the study of pain, an endeavour that began with Freud's *Project* of 1895.

Melzack (1993) discusses his and Patrick Wall's development of the concept of the "gate control theory" in 1965, however it was not presented until 1970. This concept explained the "modulation of inputs in the spinal dorsal horns and the dynamic role of the brain in pain processes. [...] Psychological factors, which were previously dismissed as 'reaction to pain', were now seen to be an integral part of pain processing." The significant contribution of this theory was that it emphasised the mechanisms of the central nervous system and to the establishment of the role of the brain as an active system that filters, selects, and modulates inputs. In his article *Pain: Past, Present and Future* Melzack explains that "the gate control theory of pain" proposes that

> a mechanism in the dorsal horns of the spinal cord acts like a gate
> which inhibits or facilitates transmission from the body to the brain
> on the basis of the diameters of the active peripheral fibers as well
> as the dynamic action of brain processes. As a result, psychological
> variables such as past experiences, attention and other cognitive

activities have been integrated into current research and therapy on pain processes. (1993, pp. 615–619)

I propose that when considering the "gate control theory" we may view "gate" as a metaphor for a defence mechanism that prevents certain unconscious memories from rising to the surface of consciousness. The "dorsal horns" controls the quality and intensity of physical pain and the body's response to external stimuli. This could be compared to the activities of the "ego" in modulating psychic pain, such as repression, in response to internal or external psychological stimuli.

The dorsal horns were, too, not merely passive transmission stations but sites at which dynamic activities—inhibitions, excitations, and modulation—occurred. Melzack and Wall, as Freud strived to achieve, acknowledged pain as the motivating factor in subjective experiences and human behaviour. They stated that there are specialised systems involved in the "sensory-discriminative, motivational-affective and evaluative dimensions of pain" (ibid., p. 619).

Pribram and Gill (1976) support Freud's *Project* further for setting up certain foundations for future research in spite of various drawbacks. They stated that:

> In the terms of the *Project*, Freud should have recognized that both pain and unpleasure are "qualitative" not "quantitative" conceptions since they are perceived in consciousness. Therefore, by his own thesis, some pattern (measurable in terms of quality or information) or lack of pattern must be responsible for the perception of pain and unpleasure—a "quantitative" energy explanation is out of place. Freud in fact recognized this but belatedly. (pp. 49–50)

Further, explanations in terms of patterning in pain and unpleasure would have left the way open for incorporating the results of subsequent research on the neurological nature of pain and its control. Research further indicates that neurons that can be excited by painful stimuli are also excited by:

> touch pressure or proprioceptive manipulations. A control process based on a negative feedback mechanism at the spinal cord level has therefore been proposed. When that control is exercised by pattern, stimulation from somatosensory receptors, touch, pressure,

etc., are perceived; when uncontrolled positive feedback produces oscillatory and disruptive stimulation, unpatterned pain is perceived. (ibid.)

In this instance, it seems that Freud was partially correct in proposing that an increase in quantity *disrupts* pattern and this *unpatterned* excitation is perceived as pain. However, "conscious awareness of pain, as is the case elsewhere, is dependent on the dimension of pattern—the lack of pattern in this case" (ibid., p. 50).

Melzack's theory of the neuromatrix

Melzack conceptualised that a unified brain mechanism "lies at the heart of the new theory" and believes the word "neuromatrix" best characterises it. He implied that the matrix was something within which something else originates and takes form. It is a widespread network of neurons in the brain that make up the "anatomical substrate of the body-self"—an imprint or map of the body-self (1993, p. 623).

The neuromatrix is a template of the whole unity of the body/self. It produces the characteristic neural pattern for the whole body—the neurosignature. It also produces subsets of signature patterns that relate to events at or in different parts of the body.

The neuromatrix is distributed throughout many areas of the brain and comprises a large widespread network of neurons, that consist of loops between the thalamus and the cortex as well as the limbic system, which, through repeated cyclical processing and synthesis, generates a characteristic pattern which is the neurosignature which ultimately produces the pattern that is felt as a whole body. Certain parts of the neuromatrix are specialised to process major sensory events such as injury, temperature change, and stimulation of erogenous tissue which impress sub-signatures on the larger neurosignature.

Individual information from the skin, joints, muscles, and so on converges to produce the experience of a coherent, articulated body. Besides this, there are millions of nerve impulses at any given time, arriving at the brain, from all of the sensory systems of the body. In the same way, a pattern or sub-signature is created for sensory impulse from injurious event. The injury, however, is *not pain.*

Pain occurs and is felt in the brain as a *quality of experience.* The qualities of experience are inherently built in to the brain and not learned.

Meaningful experiences of movement, the coordination of limbs, pain in a missing limb—all occur and are felt in the brain.

What is significant in Melzack and Wall's (1993) research is their mapping of the brain functions to explain the impact of internal and external stimuli on the body and mind. Of considerable importance is their theory that the "body-self is still present in experience even when input from that (missing) part of the body is gone" (Melzack, 1989). The spatial distribution and synaptic links are initially determined genetically and are later sculpted by sensory inputs.

These neural loops diverge to allow parallel processing in different components of this network. They also converge continually to allow interactions between the "output products of processing". This cycle of "processing and synthesis", of the nerve impulses through the neuromatrix, conveys a pattern or signature which is characteristic of these processes called the neurosignature. The signature is produced by the patterns of "synaptic connections" or nerve impulse patterns, in the entire neuromatrix. The signature is imparted on all these nerve impulse patterns that flow through the neuromatrix.

> All inputs from the body undergo cyclical processing and synthesis so that characteristic patterns are impressed on them in the neuromatrix. Portions of the neuromatrix are specialized to process information related to major sensory events (such as injury, temperature change and stimulation of erogenous tissue) and may be labelled as neuromodules which impress subsignatures on the larger neurosignature. The neurosignature, which is a continuous outflow from the body-self neuromatrix, is projected to areas in the brain—the *sentient neural hub (SNH)*—in which the stream of nerve impulses (the neurosignature modulated by ongoing inputs) is converted into a continually changing stream of awareness. (Melzack & Wall, 1993, pp. 621–622)

The neurosignature originates and takes form in the neuromatrix and though the neurosignature (nerve impulse patterns) may be triggered or modulated by input, the input is only a "trigger" and does not produce the neurosignature itself.

Melzack proposes that there are four components of this conceptual nervous system: (1) the body-self neuromatrix; (2) cyclical processing and synthesis in which the neurosignature is produced; (3) the sentient neural hub which converts (transduce) the flow of neurosignatures into the flow of awareness; and (4) activation of an action neuromatrix to provide the *pattern* of movements to bring about the desired goal or behaviour (ibid.).

The neuromatrix is the central system within the brain, where the signature of specific patterns of behaviour originates that may be triggered by stimuli to activate certain responses. There is also a "characteristic neurosignature" created within the neuromatrix, according to this theory, for the complexity of feelings experienced.

It is unimaginable how the brain processes the enormous amount of information that it receives through all its senses to create the experience of a "whole body". Melzack states that he visualises a genetically build-in neuromatrix for the whole body, producing a characteristic neurosignature of the body which carries with it patterns for the innumerable qualities we feel. It seems that the neuromatrix produces a "continuous message" as a result of its cyclical processing and synthesis. This represents the whole body in which details are "differentiated within the whole as inputs come into it" (ibid., p. 623).

Following this assumption, "pain is not injury; *the quality of pain experiences* must not be confused with the physical event" but rather "the *quality of experience* must be generated by the structures of the brain" (ibid.).

Due to the genetic nature of the creation and evolution of these imprints it is not necessary for a stimulus to be present for there to be a sense of an experience of pain or the experience of *being in pain* which can be identified as a *quality* of pain. The triggers from stimuli in turn, then, motivate action towards the satisfaction of needs, wishes, and desires. Melzack states that "the neuromatrix is a psychologically meaningful unit, developed by both heredity and learning, that represents an entire unified entity" (ibid., p. 625).

The neuromatrix unifies the body as a whole and is genetically programmed to operate a certain way—as the established neurosignatures dictate. The unconscious, I propose, is also a matrix within which lies a network of emotions and feelings similar to the neural network, as will be discussed in the next chapter.

Conclusion

Freud was able to draw up a model for the neurological system's processes in an effort to explain his psychological theory of pain processing. He discovered that the neurological system employed certain resistances and defences, via the two types of neurons, to control affect, attempting to either inhibit or excite the release of energy, causing certain actions and behaviours. He also observed that psychological trauma and physical trauma triggered a similar reaction to the experience of having pain. There appeared to be certain elements present, in the systems of the mind also, that were inhibitory or excitatory, yet he could not set this down in scientifically tangible, processes. His assumption was that similar processes as those of neuronal activity took place in the mind as well, to produce a similar reaction to stimuli.

Melzack and Wall's concept of the gate control theory implicated the psychological system, as the metaphor of the "gate" can be applied to the ego's regulatory mechanism. Melzack's (1993) further research into neurological systems brought him to an explanation of pain in the *absence* of peripheral stimuli. This, in turn brought him to his concept of the neuromatrix. This concept also takes Freud's theory of the modulation of the movement of energy through the neuronal systems, perception, memory, and motivation, and Wall's theory of the gate control theory one step further.

Freud wanted to explain further the concepts of consciousness, memory, motive, and perception within his model in the *Project* and speculated about imprinted patterns of activity within the neural network that produced reaction and behaviour. He knew that somehow this impacted on psychological processes and endeavoured to justify these within the neurological model.

Melzack's neuromatrix models a system within which all neurological experiences are imprinted, creating patterns of activity (impact, actions and reactions), which are triggered with each event. Within this matrix, there are not only neurological patterns (neurosignature), but also psychological patterns.

The one element which is clear is that pain is the *quality of experience* which is registered in the brain and the mind. On the one hand, it is a breach of either the neurobiological system or the psychological system, and on the other hand, a protective factor, as it warns against harm or distress. For example, if you place your hand on a hot burner, pain will make you quickly take your hand away, or if a loved one dies you will feel the pain of loss and grief or in other cases remorse is triggered—all aid in the process of physical or emotional healing.

Freud established that pain is a component of human development within the complexities of human relationships. His theory of pain processing and that of Melzack and Wall's is similar in that it identifies that *pain* represents a multifaceted *category* of experiences of sensory, affective and evaluative dimensions.

A component of both theories of pain processing is that experiences are imprinted in the matrices of the brain and mind. These imprints create perceptions, memories, and motives provoking impetus for either inhibiting or allowing behaviour. My argument is that memory and motive are two important components triggered by an individual's emotional *suffering* or *being in pain* (due to historical, unresolved, emotional trauma—physical and/or psychological). The continuous actions of the neurological as well as the psychological systems to maintain a certain "whole" create an environment of tensions and anxieties at subjective and varying degrees, since a "whole" is not possible. I propose that the variety of emotional imprints stored in the unconscious becomes a *conglomerate* (of pain) which collectively affects thought and behaviour throughout the subject's life. Although, each experience will have its own interpretation and manifestation when triggered by certain events the *pain of loss*, as Freud (1950a) identified, lies at the heart of being in pain or suffering. I propose that it is with this *being in pain* that the subject has a relationship and which influences how he views himself and his existence.

CHAPTER THREE

The conceptualisation of the psychomatrix and the subject-pain relationship

Introduction

In Chapter Two, I discussed Freud's 1895 theory of pain as set out in his *Project* (1950a). The theories and assumptions he discussed in this work reverberated throughout the rest of his work as he spoke about the processes of mental activity. This is particularly evident in *Beyond the Pleasure Principle* (1920g) where he posits that external stimuli powerful enough to breach the protective shield can be described as traumatic. The concept of trauma unavoidably implies that there is a connection with this kind of breach that fails to protect the organism against noxious stimuli. Such external traumas will, inevitably

> provoke a disturbance on a large scale in the functioning of the organism's energy and sets in motion every possible defensive measure. At the same time, the pleasure principle is for the moment put out of action. [...] Cathectic energy is summoned from all sides to provide sufficiently high cathexes of energy in environs of the breach. (pp. 29–30)

In the last chapter, I also discussed Melzack and Wall's theories of pain and Melzack's concept of the neuromatrix derived from further research, which began with his and Wall's "gate control theory" of pain processing. The common denominator of these pain processing systems and the subject *being in pain* is simply that pain is a multifaceted, subjective phenomenon experienced by each individual.

This chapter will examine some of Freud's major concepts to evidence the possibility of a psychomatrix which functions in tandem with the neuromatrix. Most importantly, the discussion will endeavour to lead to an understanding of the significance of the concept of the psychomatrix to the subject-pain relationship.

Freud's theory of the unconscious

Freud's theory of the unconscious holds that a wide array of human behaviour is a manifestation of what is hidden within the dimensions of the mental process—the unconscious. He treated his neurotic patients, displaying certain behaviours, from this frame of reference. Their behaviour was meaningful in that they were manifestations of the root causes of their sufferings. He believed that our words and actions were not arbitrary or illogical actions but had unconscious motives and meanings behind them. Freud (1923b) states:

> The division of the psychical into what is conscious and what is unconscious is the fundamental premise of psycho-analysis; and it alone makes it possible for psycho-analysis to understand the pathological processes in mental life, which are as common as they are important. [...] Psycho-analysis cannot situate the essence of the psychical in consciousness, but is obliged to regard consciousness as a quality of the psychical, which may be present in addition to other qualities or may be absent. (p. 13)

The unconscious has implications, then, for all human behaviour. To use a common analogy the conscious has been likened to the tip of an iceberg and what lies beneath is the unconscious complexities of the human psyche.

The instincts or drives are integral parts of the unconscious as they influence conscious behaviour. These are the motivating energies in the mental processes and human behaviour. Freud identified two main instincts—the life instinct, that influences self-preservation and sexuality, and the death instinct that influences aggression and destruction. Both work in tandem to preserve the cycle of life.

In his first topography, Freud divided the mind into three systems/ agencies—conscious (*Cs*), preconscious (*Ps*), and unconscious (*Ucs*). In the second topographical model, he creates the structure of the ego, id, and superego. Together these structures have been used to explain the complexities of the impressions and imprints of past and present of human experiences, the various and diverse levels of reactions to these and the multifaceted behaviours. These are the mechanisms that influence the processes of, and motivate, human actions and reactions to fulfilling desires, and dealing with issues in life, such as loss (Freud, 1920g, 1923b).

The unconscious is, of course, the primary concern of my book as it has significant implications in my proposal of a *psychomatrix* which, I propose, is a system that sits within the *matrix* of the unconscious. Its purpose is to synthesise the phenomenon of *pain* and its processes.

The psychomatrix

Similar to the neuromatrix, I propose that there exists a psychomatrix that behaves concurrently with the systems of the body and brain. Impressions are generated from traumatic, unconscious emotions and repressed representations of historical events that may be the psycho-signatures created in the matrix. Emotional stimuli, influenced by these signatures, then trigger conscious responses. This, I think, may also be a metaphor for Freud's (1920, 1923b) life and death instincts. As Melzack (1993) postulates, the neuromatrix is influenced by inherent qualities. Freud has posited that instincts, as well, are inherent qualities of life and death that, I suggest, in turn, may facilitate the processes within a psychomatrix.

Freud states that the two classes of instincts work for as well as against each other and that the "emergence of life would thus be the cause of the continuance of life and also at the same time the striving towards death; and life itself would be a conflict and a compromise between these two trends" (1923b, pp. 40–41).

The conflicts that Freud discusses are part and parcel of my theory of a relationship between the subject and his pain, the development of which, I propose, is inherent within the psychomatrix. I suppose that like the "dream space" the unconscious is a "space"—a space that holds representations of experiences past and present. However, this data is far from being static but dynamic as it morphs according to the processes of development and influenced by the psychosignature.

The main "nodule" (Melzack, 1993) in the psychomatrix is that of a pain signature. In metapsychological terms, it is the pain that goes beyond acute physical and psychological pain. It is the emotional suffering that influences our responses to situations and events—our day-to-day experiences. The psychosignature is that of a desire for pain and is influenced by the stimuli that are received by the psychomatrix. I propose that the unconscious is where the psychomatrix is situated and has been innately formed to synthesise the complexities and ambiguities of pain—that of suffering or "being in pain" (Pontalis, 1981). It is the emotional imprint of what is desired as well as *undesired* by the brain/ mind/body schema—pain, during a response to internal or external trauma.

From its space in the psychomatrix, pain, has a far-reaching influence on human rationale for actions and behaviours. As discussed earlier, research has begun to acknowledge the links between physical and psychological pain. It has identified mechanisms that compel processes in the brain that manipulate physical as well as psychological responses. However, the question of pain—its existence and purpose— has not been scientifically satisfactorily explained.

One thing that is clear is that after an acute event has been treated and the threat has been removed, there continues to be pain in varying degrees that lives a complex life in the emotional sphere. I suppose that the impression which is left behind is a stimulus that passes through the psychomatrix where it is influenced and reorganised by the psychosignature which triggers past, emotional and unresolved traumas. Although what is triggered is not *expressed* in such *language,* it is *felt* within the emotional system of the psychomatrix. This, I propose, is the *being in pain or suffering*—desire for the lost object and a sense of unity— which influences thoughts and behaviour.

The response or output from the psychomatrix then, is behaviour or actions towards the aim of maintaining a certain circumstance or situation. Or, even to maintain an environment that attracts or provokes certain external reactions therefore, creating within the subject a sense of satisfaction or pleasure. There are a variety of scenarios that may evidence this statement. However, the ones that I have encountered most often, in the course of my work, are those of chronic pain, addictions, and phantom limb syndrome which will be discussed in subsequent chapters. Gamsa's (1993) statement that "the view that emotional states generate or exacerbate pain has a long history" is a simple statement but with complex implications for the problem of pain (p. 5).

Various scientists, such as Merskey (1965, 1985), Merskey and Spear (1967), Szasz (1957), Melzack and Wall (1965, 1996, 1993), and Melzack (1993, 2006) have endeavoured to answer the question, "How can there be pain if pain and organs are not being stimulated?" (Gamsa, 1993, p. 6). Gamsa writes that further research by Engel in 1959 offered a developmental theory to explain "psychogenic" pain, that is, pain in the absence of peripheral stimulation. From the time of birth, in Engel's view, the individual builds a "library" of pain experiences, originating from (and associated with) pain provoked by peripheral stimulation. Engel postulates that throughout our developmental stages, pain acquires meaning contingent upon the context within which it occurs. This meaning may later become a trigger or triggers for pain without peripheral stimulation. For example, a baby's cry draws attention which in turn brings comfort from the mother and thus, pain becomes a cue for reunion with a love object. In early childhood, pain is also directly linked with punishment which in turn serves to expiate guilt.

> From these early associations, some individuals come to use pain unconsciously to resolve developmental conflicts and to restore psychic balance. These early psychodynamics contribute to the development of "pain-prone" disorder, with the following characteristics: a) conscious and unconscious guilt with pain serving as atonement; b) a history of suffering, defeat, and intolerance of success, suggesting a masochistic character structure; c) a strong unfulfilled aggressive drive, with pain substituting for aggression; and d) development of pain to replace feelings of loss or fear of threatened loss of a relationship. (ibid., p. 7)

My question, then, is what is this "library" that Engel speaks about? I propose that it is the psychomatrix and where the psychosignature of pain is created. However, I make a further speculation that the psychomatrix is innate and an integral part of our genetic make-up. In the spirit of Freud's interest in Darwin, I would like to venture that one's specific, psychic, genetic make-up can imply the development of the psychosignature. For example, if we research and discover what our great-grandmother or great-grandfather was like, as far as dealing with certain situations in their lives, we may get a good explanation of the evolution of our own responses to our present circumstances. The experiences that become imprints or impressions within the psychomatrix, from birth, add to the subjectivity of our specific pain psychosignature. The "library" scenario then is valid as it also implies that the content is accessible to the subject mediated by internal and external, situational stimuli. However, the input is then influenced or modulated by the psychosignature, leaving the possibility that this causes the output of behaviour to be modified by this process.

There are certain phenomena that cannot, at present, be explained in scientific terms as Freud discovered even then, with his 1895 *Project* (1950a). He put these phenomena down to metapsychological events. The creation of his structures of the mind to explain levels of consciousness and entities that influence mental and physical behaviour is a clear indication of his idea of metapsychology. This gave him the frame of reference that he needed to work, so effectively, from as he, at the same time, set the foundations for further research into the links between the processes of the brain and the mind. One of these was the nature of memory. Sacks (1998) states that Freud:

> saw memory as central in hysteria (*"hysterics suffer mainly from reminiscences"*); and in the Project he attempted to explicate the physiological basis of memory at many levels. One physiological prerequisite for memory, he postulated, was a system of "contact barriers" between certain neurons—his so-called psi system (this was a decade before Sherrington gave synapses their name). Freud's contact barriers were capable of selective facilitation or inhibition, thus allowing permanent neuronal changes which corresponded to the acquisition of new information and new memories [...]. At a higher level, Freud regarded memory and motives as inseparable. (p. 19)

He posited that recollections would have no significance unless associated with motives. Freud's theory took memory far beyond the "local neuronal traces". To him memories were primarily a dynamic, transforming and reorganising force throughout life. The influence of memory was the core within the formation of identity and "nothing more guaranteed one's continuity as an individual". However, due to the reorganising capacity of memories, "no one was more sensitive than Freud to the reconstructive potential of memory, the fact that memories are continually worked over and that their essence, indeed, *is* recategorization" (ibid.).

The dynamic nature of memories is essential to the capacity of an individual to change or alter his behaviour. However, the integral piece of the puzzle to giving memory its quality is pain—the emotional suffering that is the make-up of the psychosignature. I propose that a memory is a stimulus that enters the psychomatrix to then be modulated and re-categorised by the psychosignature. This would then give it the quality it needs to influence behaviour. Another key point that Sacks (1998) makes is that "the potential for therapy, for change, therefore lies in the capacity to exhume such 'fixated' material into the present so that it can be subjected to the creative process of *retranscription* and thus allow the stalled individual to grow once again and change" (ibid., p. 20; my italics).

As we can see, pain is a prominent figure in the subject's life and is pervasive throughout all domains of existence and influences our very identity, thus my theory that there is a distinct possibility of the existence of a psychomatrix in the service of the subject-pain relationship.

Consider this question—which is not a new question, but one that has been asked by greater thinkers in a variety of ways: Is there a possibility that there exists a fear, in some, of losing the ability to feel good, if they feel bad for too long, and in others, a need to feeling bad for fear that feeling good takes them to feeling a bad that they could not, emotionally, deal with? This, I believe, speaks to the fear of either acknowledging that pain is necessary to one's life for fear of knowing nothing else or a fear of feeling only pleasure and losing sight of purpose. This is a significant aspect within the subject-pain relationship and one that the subject struggles with throughout life.

A vast spectrum of (ongoing) research has identified the impact of cultural, religious, social, and political factors on pain and pain management. I will argue that all of these figure in the conglomerate that I call *pain*. Considering the meaning of pain in one's life, there exists the possibility of a relationship between the subject and the pain that he experiences, consciously and unconsciously. Pain becomes an object that compels the subject to respond accordingly and consequently. These manifestations have an impact not only on his life but also on his surrounding environment.

There are other recent studies, that evidence the influence and serious impact of psychological and emotional pain on an individual's life, and that psychological distress presents as an obstacle to recovery for patients. For example, a study conducted by Hall et al. (2011, p. 1049) indicated that psychological distress impacts on long-term disability consistently and showed that "depression and stress individually were both partial mediators in the pain-disability relationship. Therefore, pain measured at six weeks after the onset of pain indirectly affects future disability by influencing symptoms of depression and symptoms of stress." It goes on to explain that anxiety plays a major role as its affects psychological processes and was indicated as a mechanism to explain how (psychological and emotional) pain leads to subsequent disabilities. One's relationship with pain will influence how he reacts to having pain and the decisions as to how to manage this *having pain*. In doing, so as in the scenario above, one may "use" *having pain* as a motive toward fulfilling a means of managing certain life conditions and perpetuating an environment which may promote their physical condition to that end. The dichotomy is that for the subject the *being in pain* or *suffering* will also continue unhampered.

Loss, perversion and narcissism

Pain enters an individual's life when he experiences loss of an object that he is attached to. For the sake of this argument I refer to Schore (2001, p. 429) regarding his theory on attachment:

> ... in forming an attachment bond of somatically expressed emotional communications, the mother is synchronizing and resonating with the rhythms of the infant's dynamic internal states and then regulating the arousal level of these negative and positive states. Attachment is thus the dyadic (interactive) regulation of emotion (Sroufe, 1996). [...] attachment is more than overt behaviour, it is internal, being built into the nervous system, in the course and as a result of the infant's experience of his transactions with the mother. (Ainsworth, 1967, p. 429) (Schore, 2001, p. 307)

I think this further explains, scientifically, the rationale for trauma of loss of the object. It is also an indication of the relational sphere of the subject's perception to the (anxiety) pain which he experiences. According to this theory and others' such as Bowlby (1969, 1978), the mother is key in creating a safe and secure environment for the infant to grow and mature. One of the main developmental domains is learning how to deal with loss. As Schore (2001) states: "Regulated interactions with a familiar predictable primary caregiver create not only a sense of safety, but also a positively charged curiosity that fuels the burgeoning self's exploration of novel socioemotional and physical environments".

The experiences of childhood, when we speak about loss, are at best traumatic—whether or not there has been a healthy attachment to the (object) mother. The impact of these experiences comes in subjective and varying degrees. The reaction to loss is pain. The realisation, following the acute event of loss or the losing of "the object", that there is an emptiness or void, is when emotional suffering begins. Loss of the womb, loss of the breast, the lack of satisfaction of instincts, and later the loss of the mother, the first love object, leaves a lasting impact (Freud, 1905d). As Freud (1926d discussed, loss of the object can provoke pain, which is part of mourning and anxiety.

The infant plays a passive part on the one hand; however, on the other, he is active, to some degree, in situating his own body and finding satisfaction in an object apart from the breast. However, the development stages prove to be a challenge as the element of loss introduces itself in many guises. Behaviours that ensue as a result of loss and pain are complex as has been established throughout past and present research. A group of behaviours that is most pertinent to this investigation is found in what Freud (1905d, 1920g) has labelled as perverse. Since then, there has been much research that has gone into the definition of this complex subject.

In exploring the psychoanalytic perspectives on "loss", it is clear that loss—translated as "cut", "void", "emptiness"—causes pain. I propose that this empty space is where an individual feels a sense of annihilation. The acute impact of the initial "castration" is felt as shock— a paralysis that eventually gives way to the feelings of being in pain (Freud, 1905d, 1920g, 1926d; Pontalis, 1981; Stoller, 1991; Gamsa, 1994).

I further venture to theorise that during this phase of paralysis, a stimulus has reached the psychomatrix—and the output of behaviour, in its many varieties carries the impact of pain within. The pain suffered by the individual, which is a subjective response, is what motivates his behaviour and actions.

In Freud's (1920g) famous example of a child at play making sounds that were expressions taken as representing the German words *fort* (gone) and *da* (there), with a wooden reel and a piece of string Freud discusses this an acting-out of loss and emptiness. He states that the child played the first half of the game most of the time—where he throws it away. But at times, he would also carry the game out through to the second half where he pulls it back. This is a repetition of a traumatic event where his mother had left him for the first time. Apparently, he survived the mother leaving without fuss—as many children do (not all, of course, as there are those who cry out in protest of being left). However, the *not crying*, I suggest, is the child being in shock. The behaviour that comes forth following this is an indication of his sense of loss and his need to overcome the feelings of loss. Throwing the object away— waiting a moment—then pulling it back. But, as has been mentioned— most of the time he just threw the object away seemingly not interested in completing the action.

It appears to be an aggressive action. He throws it away and awaits its "reaction"—then pulls it back not giving it an opportunity to react— so to speak. He throws it into the empty "space" so as to make it experience the same pain that he is in. Then pulls it back in an effort to show his "mastery" over the "object" (his mother), and its actions, as well as control over his own actions. He is in control. The pleasure in the repetitive behaviour, in the first place, is knowing that he has actively overcome his loss. And, secondly, to show that he does not have to be a "passive object" to the (object of desire) mother (Freud, 1920g, pp. 14–17).

Another aspect of loss is the "breach" in the protective shield that Freud (ibid., pp. 29–30) speaks about—whether it is a breach in the protective psychological or physical shield. Our sense of security and safety is challenged and breached. I propose that every breach is a form of loss, as we lose a part of this sense of security. The breach is a stimulus that reaches the psychomatrix where it is influenced by the psychosignature of pain within, adding to the impressions already within. The response is in the form of anxiety.

We strive to defend ourselves from these anxieties and the pain of a sense of loss. The patterns of behaviour indicate that our reaction to this unpleasure is to seek out the opposite—pleasure. Freud stressed this certain human preoccupation of seeking pleasure throughout his work, particularly in *The Pleasure Principle* and *Beyond the Pleasure Principle* (1920g). Before pleasure is achieved, though, reality has a way of presenting itself. However, this does not dampen the desire for achieving pleasure indeed it may even exacerbate the need for it.

The human capacity to derive pleasure in the face of pain has been of interest not only to Freud but, also to other researchers in the field, to explain the existence of pain. In *Mourning and Melancholia* (1917e), Freud's explanation of melancholia is of interest to my work, as the complexities of the presence of pain and pleasure (as are love and hate) are clearly identified in his explanation of melancholia:

> This conflict of ambivalence, now more real, now more constitutive in origin, should not be neglected among the preconditions of melancholia. If the love of the object, which cannot be abandoned while the object itself is abandoned, has fled into narcissistic identification, hatred goes to work on this substitute object, insulting it, humiliating it, making it suffer and deriving a sadistic satisfaction from that suffering. The indubitably pleasurable self-torment of melancholia, like the corresponding phenomenon of obsessive neurosis, signifies the satisfaction of tendencies of sadism and hatred, which are applied to an object and are thus turned back against the patient's own person. In both of these illnesses, patients manage to avenge themselves on the original objects along the detour of self-punishment, and to torment their loved ones by means of being ill, having taken to illness in order to avoid showing their hostility directly. (2005, p. 211)

Human beings are very creative in finding compensatory ways in which they can derive pleasure while still dealing with the reality of a traumatic or difficult situation. For example, if a baby is hungry and food is not ready instantly he sucks his thumb or he cries (Freud, 1905d, pp. 180–182). To cope with a limb that has been amputated the brain will create a "phantom limb" which makes itself known in the form of pain (derived from Ramachandran, 1998), or mourning the death of a loved one (Freud, 2005).

Loss of the object implicates the many challenges of the developmental stages. From what has been discussed so far, it seems that these are not just challenges but, can present insurmountable obstacles to living a productive life in the normal sense that society has created. Losing the safety and security of the mother (object)—from the trauma of birth and the cutting of the umbilical cord to the breast—leaves an everlasting impression. The desire to "re-find" the object is the culprit in the many diverse and complex patterns of human behaviour. While striving to achieve the aims of this primary pleasure (being part of the object in the womb or at the breast) the subject engages in many, complex behaviours that could, at times, be labelled as perverse. Stoller (1991) agrees with Freud (1905d) when he states that "the 'perversions' are not entities but simply behaviours in which all kinds of folks indulge" (p. 36).

Freud (1905d) postulates that aggressiveness and a desire to *conquer* is a usual element in most men therefore, sadism would be a link to the "aggressive component of the sexual instinct". He continues to explain that in day to day language the connotation of sadism oscillates between being characterised by an active or violent attitude toward the sexual object, and where satisfaction is entirely "conditional on the humiliation and maltreatment of the object". It is only the later extreme which "deserves to be described as a perversion" (pp. 157–158).

Freud has said that "perversions are sexual activities which either (a) extend, in an anatomical sense, beyond the regions of the body that are designed for sexual union, or (b) linger over the intermediate relations to the sexual object which should normally be traversed rapidly on the path towards the final sexual aim" (1905d, p. 150).

Further research has offered several perspectives on perversions. In exploring the work of several researchers in the field of psychoanalysis, Cooper (1991) has identified that the common denominators appear to be loss (connoting a circumstance resulting from a forced "taking away" of something), abandonment, rejection, and loss of control where an individual feels a sense of helplessness (forced to be in a passive position), and a threat to life (a sense of annihilation). He states that Stoller (1974) "melds the concept of sexuality and the older emphasis on castration and fetishism in forming a perversion with newer concepts derived from the understanding of preoedipal narcissistic and safety needs and the problem of separation and individuation" (pp. 20–21).

Stoller (1991) explains his views on perversion stating that perversion is the erotic form of hatred and usually a fantasy usually acted on but "occasionally restricted to a daydream" either one's own creation or based on others' creations such as, pornography.

> It is a habitual, preferred aberration necessary for one's full satisfaction, primarily motivated by hostility. By *hostility* I mean a state in which one wishes to harm an object; that differentiates it from *aggression*, which often implies only forcefulness. The hostility in

perversion takes form in a fantasy of revenge hidden in the actions that make up the perversion and serves to convert childhood trauma to adult triumph. To create the greatest excitement, the perversion must also portray itself as an act of risk taking. (1991, p. 37)

In other words, *sin*. That is, excitement comes from an awareness—conscious or unconscious—that one is harming, *needs* to harm, *wants* to harm. More precisely, the harm done is an act of humiliating in revenge for one's having been humiliated (ibid.).

I propose that "hatred" embodies "fear"—fear of loss, of security and a fear of annihilation. Fear is an experience of pain as it encompasses anxiety of the known as well as the unknown (Kierkegaard, in Hong & Hong, 2000, pp. 138–139). The fear (pain) can be traced back to the infantile stage and to the "loss of the object" (Freud, 1905d, 1914c, 1920g, 1926d).

According to Stoller's (1991) argument above, the fantasy plays a key role in the desire to regain the subject's control and sense of power. It is a space where the subject can be omnipotent in fulfilling his desires. It is an internal, narcissistic space where he has withdrawn his libido, in part, to the ego. Within this state of "self-love" there is the need for "self-preservation". It has features of the preoedipal stage of development where the loss of the object has been the primary source of pain. It is however, not only the need for self-preservation but also a pathological need to destroy the object that has caused this breach in his "protective shield" (Freud, 1920g). The protective shield, in this case, being his sense of omnipotence, where his every basic need (desire for pleasure) is fulfilled. The breach causes a narcissistic concentration of all his attention (energy) on his ego where the pain is being experienced (Freud, 1920g, p. 30).

The awareness of loss tends to give the subject a sense of isolation and separation from the external world, accompanied by a sense of helplessness. In his paper, *On Narcissism: An Introduction* (1914c), Freud states:

The libido that has been withdrawn from the external world has been directed to the ego and thus gives rise to an attitude which may be called narcissism. [...] a person who is tormented by organic pain and discomfort gives up his interest in the things of the external world, in so far as they do not concern his suffering.

> Closer observation teaches us that he also withdraws libidinal interest from his love-objects: so long as he suffers he ceases to love. (pp. 75–82)

However, once the pain abates the libido gradually, once more, returns to the external world and its objects (ibid., p. 82).

At the stage of primary narcissism the desire for self-preservation contains not only the ego libido, but this libido flows into the parallel system of the sexual libido. The sexual instinct and that of nourishment at this point have not been differentiated. The infant is absorbed in experiencing pleasure from the object (breast/mother) that he identifies with as part of himself. In the object's absence, he discovers that he can derive the same pleasure and satisfaction within a perfunctory awareness (autoeroticism) of his own body. In this process, however, he begins to realise that the object is not a part of his own body, but an object apart, and one that he is dependent upon for fulfilment of needs. The sense of separation is painful yet necessary in the further development of object choice (Treurniet, 1991).

Freud (1905d) postulates: "The satisfaction of the erotogenic zone is associated in the first instance, with the satisfaction of the need for nourishment. To begin with, sexual activity attaches itself to functions serving the purpose of self-preservation and does not become independent of them until later" (pp. 181–182). Primary narcissism is then the libidinal investment of the self and is part and parcel of normal early development. Even during the process of development, in the investment in external objects, part of this narcissism is retained in the unconscious. It becomes a mechanism in the development of self-esteem and self-regard (Freud, 1914c).

In contrast to primary narcissism is the mechanism of secondary narcissism which arises in pathological states. The subject withdraws its libido from the external world in a re-investment of the self.

> This happens especially in cases of disappointment with the object or in mourning for a lost object; further, it occurs as a normal developmental process in secondary identification and where some of the libidinal investment of the admired or loved object is then transferred to the self as a consequence of this identification. Finally, it also happens when a person lives up to his ideals. (Treurniet, 1991, p. 79)

The development of the ego plays a primary role in the development of the subject's sense of self, which evolves through the stage of infancy and early childhood. The development of the ego-ideal (conscience) to which it is accountable is essential in establishing its ideals (Freud, 1914).

The pathological dimension of secondary narcissism manifests in the complexities of perversion. A withdrawal of the libido from external investment, as I have discussed above, is a pathological state and arises out of a traumatic impact. An essential component of primary narcissism is the transition from ego libido to object libido and secondary identification that implicates the relation of the subject to the object. In encountering the castration complex a most significant psychic event occurs impacting on the subject's development. At this point ego instincts and libidinal instinct remain undifferentiated and the subject's anxieties are focused on his own person—and the "cut" or "void".

Cooper (1991) explains:

> the narcissistic base of perverse development I want to emphasize is that the core trauma in many if not all perversions is the experience of terrifying passivity in relation to the preoedipal mother perceived as dangerously malignant, malicious, and all-powerful, arousing sensations of awe and the uncanny. The development of a perversion is a miscarried repair of this injury, basically through dehumanization of the body and the construction of three core fantasies designed to undo the intolerable sense of helplessness. Stoller and Khan have taught us about dehumanization in perversion and its relation to fetishism [...]. Dehumanization is the ultimate strategy against the fear of human qualities—it protects against the vulnerability of loving, against the possibility of human unpredictability, and against the sense of powerlessness and passivity in comparison to other humans. (pp. 23–24)

The elements of sadism are, of course, what has brought this pathological but interesting, developmental dimension to attention. Sadistic tendencies, according to psychoanalytic, theory have an evolutionary aspect that runs through human development and is driven by the instincts of life and death (Freud, 1905d).

We see here that perversions are a way to manage the trauma of loss which embodies pain and all the complexities therein. Within the many levels and dimensions of masochism and sadism, we see clearly the subject-pain relational phenomenon. Pain here is present as a facilitator of gaining that which is desired—pleasure. However, once pleasure is obtained the cycle of desiring pain for more and more pleasure repeats itself to no end. Even though aspects of this cycle of pain are part of human instincts there may become exacerbated and perpetuated by the many complexities of life's processes.

Life instinct and death instinct

Freud (1920g) describes an instinct as "an urge inherent in organic life to restore an earlier state of things". He further says that "all instincts tend toward the restoration of an earlier state of things" (pp. 36–37).

Take, for example, in primary narcissism the subject's need to fulfil his desires. It is his wish to remain in a constant state of pleasure. The loss of the object is a signal that this state has been disturbed and so, fear and anxiety arise until an "earlier state of things" has been restored.

I put forward my speculations that it appears that pain in the form of conflict within the instincts is a fundamental element in the survival of human beings. Pain, enables one to know the limits of his existence. And further, that destruction and re-construction need each other to create, preserve, destroy, and recreate life in a continuous repetition of cycles. From here there appears to be a bi-polarity to every element, characteristic, and personality within human beings. By this I mean that the human condition is a composite of what exists at the extreme ends of the scale of what we (society) have come to judge as "abnormal"—a scale similar to the bi-polarity of extreme or psychotic depression and mania. Somewhere in between is what may be considered as "normal". At either end there is the experience of an utter loss of control and being detached from both identity and existence. In this powerless and mean-ingless state one engages in meaningless behaviour.

The circumstance and experiences of one's early developmental stages of life shape ones thoughts and behaviours and where one finds oneself on this bi-polar scale. It is from here that one begins to formulate an understanding of one's identity and existence and where personality and character emerge. Psychoanalytically speaking it is from here that we can begin to investigate not only the pleasure principle, whose aim is pleasure, but also the reduction of pain. This is influenced by the reality principle, but also what is beyond the pleasure principle, pain, which is influenced by the death instinct. The compulsion to repeat and master the sense of loss and annihilation is an aspect of the death instinct played out in perversion. The death instinct works in tandem with the life instinct and modified by it. Both aim to preserve life by striving to regain an earlier state of being (Freud, 1920g).

Significant elements driving the instincts are what Freud called the primary and secondary processes. The primary processes are the primary psychical processes that are unconscious. These are where desire, drive, pain, unpleasure, and the initial production of affect and wish are created, as described in the 1895 *Project* (1950a). These processes lead to a discharge of excitation. Internal and external stimuli apply their pressures on the psychical system which, in turn, result in the secondary processes being activated. The secondary processes are then the behavioural outputs from this stimulation driven by wishes of the primary processes. The secondary process is based on a memory-motive structure, within which is the desire for satisfaction, later becoming a significant element in Freud's theory of the pleasure principle, (1920g). The behaviour is, however, harnessed by the executive ego (Pribram & Gill, 1976, pp. 38–59).

Freud proposed that the aim of the *pleasure principle* is to work toward keeping an equilibrium between desire and satisfaction, "to free the mental apparatus entirely from excitation or to keep the amount of excitation in it constant or to keep it as low as possible". In other words, to "return to the quiescence of the inorganic world":

> The unbound or primary processes give rise to far more intense feelings in both directions than the bound or secondary ones. Moreover the primary processes are the earlier in time; at the beginning of mental life there are no others, and we may infer that if the pleasure principle had not already been operative in them it could never have been established for the later ones. [...] the dominance of the pleasure principle [...] has no more escaped the process of taming than other instincts in general. (1920g, pp. 63–64)

And further according to Freud, the feeling of pleasure or unpleasure is also present in the secondary process. What is pertinent to my investigation is his statement, in the same text, that, "consciousness communicates to us feelings from within not only of pleasure and unpleasure but also of a peculiar tension which in its turn can be either pleasurable or unpleasurable" (ibid). I propose that this is part of the psychosignature that would, indeed, colour the quality and quantity of the cathexis. My supposition extends further to state that the creation of the psychomatrix system is a dimension of the memory-motive structure as well as the primary and secondary processes of the systems of the mind.

Even though the aim of the life instinct is to realise the desire for pleasure, the pleasure principle serves the death instinct which is a constant sentry guarding "against increases of stimulation from within, which would make the task of living more difficult" (ibid.). This of course implicates the continuous struggle and play between the two instincts and the fulfilment of desire. All the while, the object-pain relationship is played out within the emotive desire for pain—and pleasure.

Defining subject, relationship, identity, existence, and pain

The subject is one who is seeking to attain that which he has lost. He is striving to realise his true self. He is not yet a complete "self" due to his loss. The loss which he has experienced is the loss of his primary object that was initially looked upon and believed to be one and the same entity.

I suggest that the concept of "self" is a sense of worthiness and is based first of all on primary narcissism, as Freud (1930a) discusses, which leaves residues within our character and is never destroyed; second, on how well one lives up to one's ideals (this has sociological implications within the wider community and locating one's self within it); and third, on our relationships with others and their reciprocity.

Pontalis (1981) hypothesised:

> The Freudian "subject" is defined from the outset as a series of places which are functionally specialised: this specialisation is seen in the first topography (differentiating the three systems Ucs, Pcs, Cs) as a succession, with the energy following a certain temporal *path, progredient or regredient* according to the *order* of systems. In the second topography, it is seen as an interlocking (the ego is differentiated from the id, the superego, embedded in the id, is differentiated from the ego etc.). (p. 132)

Freud created the imaginary "psychic apparatus", "to make the complications of mental functioning intelligible, by dissecting the function and assigning its different constituents to different component parts of the apparatus" (ibid.). The ego is the representation of bodily sensations from internal and external stimuli. It depends on its awareness of the body. The self is derived from identification to external objects, but separate from the object. The subject, then, is the space within which is the interplay of ego and self (ibid.).

My supposition is that the ego strives to regulate the self, as it seeks to find—re-find—the object. Initially, the infant is aware only of him "self" within a narcissistic realm of libidinal, self-preservation. His body is the source of selfish pleasure and gratification. The object is a part of this self. The process of the object becoming a separate entity is also the process by which the ego comes into play as it regulates the self and its needs to seek the object of pleasure. The self is the impoverished sense of the object as its fate is to be slave to the pleasure principle (Freud, 1920g, 1905d; Pontalis, 1981).

The notion of the self as a "space" (Pontalis, 1981) leaves it open to a speculation that the subject is left seeking to fulfil a "void" left by the object. Therefore, as Pontalis postulated, "its fate is to be slave to the pleasure principle", and constant desire to find pleasure within pain. Thus, the "self" and the "subject" are intertwined in the desire to find— re-find—the object.

Relationships, Freud stated, are what cause man the greatest pain. Humans begin with a narcissistic relationship to themselves gradually extending this to the outside world. It is the connection, bond, or attachment that one develops between self and other. The issue of relationships and the many emotional layers, within the conscious and unconscious, and the questions of human sexuality, identity, and existence, is the phenomenon of analysis (Freud, 1930a, p. 86).

Identification is based on our relations to others and as Freud (1921c) states, it is "the earliest expression of an emotional tie with another person. It plays a part in the early history of the Oedipus complex" (p. 105).

The Oedipus complex is implicated in early childhood development and influences the subject's identity and relationships throughout his life. It is an experiential process where a child develops an erotic attachment to one parent and hostility toward the other parent. There is an emotional tension that emerges within this process that is the key element in the psychic development of the subject. Here enters the "castration anxiety" for the male child, where the father is seen as an obstacle (as well as the law against incest) and presents a threat to his person in the form of castration. With the dissolution of the Oedipus complex, this desire for the mother is repressed. The female child on the other hand perceives herself as lacking the penis. Her attraction to her father is invoked by her desire to possess the penis. It is a hostile desire to take her mother's place. The dissolution of the Oedipus complex could mean the strengthening of the female child's identification with the mother (Freud, 1920g, 1923b).

Again, we see an evolutionary process take place in the development of identity. It is contingent upon one's relationship with the other, which is part of the conglomerate of pain. As explained earlier, this conglomerate is a diverse set of experiences imprinted on the matrix of the unconscious. Psychoanalysis has explained away the multi-layered processes and mechanisms at work within the creation of identities. Identity is part and parcel of our relationships with others in our personal sphere as well as the wider sphere of community. Identity is crucial to the development of the self as an endeavour to find meaning in one's existence within the complexities of his relations to others.

The narcissistic preoccupation of the self, in the form of hostility and fear of castration, comes into play within the perversions. This is a state where the subject has developed a hostile fixation on fear of his passive position in relation to the object. Namely, the mother, to the infantile lost object, which he was deprived of. Earlier, I described Stoller's (1991) perspective on perversion that explains this element.

The definition of relationship is, first of all, that it is a human characteristic. Human beings cannot but live in states of relatedness. It is the emotional dimension of the self that connects us, not only to each other, but also to the many entities in our lives. As sexual beings, we locate our identities and existence through our relationships right from the beginning of our lives (Freud, 1950a, 1905e, 1920g, 1926d, 1930a; Pontalis, 1981; Sacks, 1998). Sacks (1998) postulated:

> … remembering, for Freud, though it required such local neuronal traces (of the sort we now call long-term potentiation), went far beyond them, and was essentially dynamic, transforming, reorganizing, throughout the course of life. Nothing was more central for

the formation of identity than the power of memory; nothing more guaranteed one's continuity as an individual. (p. 19)

I have, by now, discussed the notion of *pain* throughout this investigation. Pain is based on the loss of the object, and the complexities of the re-finding of the object—the trauma of desire to fill our need for pleasure. There is an element of narcissism in this desire, as it emanates from the instinct of self-preservation as well as from object-choice and object-love (Freud, 1914c). The subject's relationship to pain can be defined upon consideration of the development of pain.

Out of the trauma to resolve the loss, which spans back to the infantile and most impressive stage of development, arise perversions, which I have discussed earlier. There is an element that could arise within the perversions, which is in the form of a fetish object, which justifies the castration complex and the post-Oedipal stage of development. A fetish object is created out of the child's fear of castration. It maintains the disavowal of the woman's penis and creates a substitute for it in another part of the woman's body. This could extend to other objects that represent the substituted object and waylay the fear of castration.

The fetish object achieves the aim of overcoming the fear of castration but also protection against it. However, on the other hand it remains a traumatic reminder of this fear and is manifested throughout the subject's life (Freud, 1927e, p. 154).

The fear of this traumatic development sets up barriers to the fulfilment of desire. This fetish object is incorporated within the desire of the object. However, the reminder of the anxiety pain of castration proves it to be unfulfilling. The fetish can be an ingredient in a perversion—the perversion being the central focus of a subject's life. The development of both has the fear of castration and pain at its root. The depth of the meaning in the fetish object is overcoming loss, rejection, humiliation, and terror of childhood (Kaplan, 1991, p. 130).

Acknowledging that at the base of the development of a fetish as well as perversion is pain I propose, that pain is the most prominent of all features within this process. From this stand point pain remains attached to all behaviour. I further propose that pain, which is caused by loss manifests in all our thoughts and actions. The experiences of pain, within fears and anxieties, are imprinted on the system of the psychomatrix. Here the pain psychosignature modifies internal and external inputs and acts in conjunction with the parallel neurological systems of the subject. Perversion and fetishism are both mechanisms influenced by pain which are modified by the psychosignature.

I propose that the phenomenon of pain within this process acts in such a way that its absence would paralyse the mental functions of the subject. The function would be depleted of its most essential and energetic motivation. If the subject suddenly lost the sense of his fetish, considering the circumstances under which it was created, he would become paralysed from his capacity to function *normally*. If the pervert lost his fantasy, the space within which he overcame the trauma of his loss and humiliation, he would be paralysed from his *normal* functioning. In both instances a breach in the protective shield, that inhibits the formation of the fetish and the fantasy, would cause a sense of loss of reality. This would surely result in a state of illness.

Pain, I suggest, is such an entity which is needed to function in the *normal* sphere of the subject's life. Pain, in other words, is a psychical object that is developed in the matrix of the psychological system, at least, as early as the primary narcissistic stage of development. It is this object that needs to be present in order for the subject to know the desire of pleasure. Therefore, the subject primarily desires pain.

Having said this, pain remains an unexplained phenomenon that has eluded specific identification. Yet, we see the many faces of it as we traverse through life. The neurology and psychology of the impact of an acute event, which causes an expression of pain, has been researched and explained by scientists such as Freud (1895), Pribram and Gill (1976), Merskey (1965, 1985), Merskey and Spear (1967), Melzack and Wall (1965, 1993), Gamsa (1993), Solms (1998), Ramachandran (1998), Schore (2001), and countless others. However, it persists in a diverse, complex, and multidimensional space within the subject and the self of being human.

Pleasure comes and goes yet pain remains faithful to the subject and his desire throughout his life. Pain sits in the void created by the subject's loss.

Conclusion

I propose that pain remains in the emotional sphere of the psychomatrix, even after the physical healing process of the body is complete and or the acute trauma has passed. This is due to how it is synthesised and modulated in the psychomatrix, by the *pain* psychosignature. There, it continues to influence thought and behaviour. It remains within the psychomatrix as a "phantom" of that acute event or experience.

I further propose that just as a limb that has been lost continues to *exist* within the body/self matrix, the sense of self, identity, relationships, and existence continue to *exist* in the matrix of the mind—beyond the trauma. Here pain maintains the unity and fidelity to the pain of loss and desire for pleasure—or the return to a state of equilibrium.

Loss and desire, for re-finding the object, translate to the conglomerate of psychological and emotional pain. It is a "cut" and a "void" that the subject, interminably, seeks to fulfil, throughout the development of his life.

The next chapter will begin the case studies which will illustrate and evidence my theory of the psychomatrix which is based on the neuromatrix described by Melzack. Freud's speculations about the similarities and links between neurological and psychological pain are fundamental to my theses of the development of the phenomenon of the subjects-pain relationship. I propose therefore, that when one enters an analytic relationship it is, inevitably, to make sense of one's relationship to pain and to understand why one's thoughts and behaviours are contingent upon one's unconscious desires to fulfil one's needs, which are based on the many aspects of one's sexuality—whether it is procreation, sustenance, or survival—it comes down to finding—re-finding—the lost object. The subject is in an interminable relationship with his (being in) *pain* as it is the *object* that he desires in order to fulfil his desires—for pleasure.

CHAPTER FOUR

The phantom limb syndrome

Introduction

The scenario of the "phantom limb" phenomenon is significant in relation to my topic. It is a metaphor for the subject's relationship with pain as I speak of it in this book. Emotional and psychological pain is comprised of the imprints of experiences that an individual has from the moment he becomes a living, breathing entity.

The concept of the "phantom" is an essential characteristic of the subject's experience—that is, its phenomenology. I propose that the value of the metaphor lies in the semantics of pain and how the subject relates to its meaning. The use of phantom pain as a metaphor describes some aspects of disembodied pain. It suggests an opening of a metaphysical or a meta-psychological conduit into another space, a space not shared with the everyday space we normally inhabit, a space that we cannot directly reach, something like an itch under the skin that you just can't get at, or an itch in the phantom limb that can be relieved only by scratching a spot on the cheek! (Ramachandran & Blakeslee, 1998, p. 29). Nonetheless, this is a space which has its own internal level and form of existence—for example, a phantom pain may have position, extent, and location on the phantom limb; or a chronic anxiety (psychological/emotional pain) may have position, extent, and location on the lower back that, otherwise, has no organic, physical diagnosis.

It is in this sense, in the context of spatiality, that I use the phantom limb phenomenon as a metaphor. In this context as well, the phantom limb syndrome has much in common with other chronic pain syndromes. When considering pain without an apparent reason I suggest, we must consider that there is the possibility of the existence of a psychomatrix in the psychological and emotional realm, parallel to Melzack's (1993) concept of the neuromatrix of the neurological system in the brain. Meanings of experiences, even though created in the mind within its subjective realm, are derived from the common meanings of words. The value of metaphor, such as the phantom limb, is that it takes the common understanding of the meanings of words (concepts) and associates it with a concept that is not so commonly understood thereby introducing a new meaning (Grey, 2000; Modell, 2003).

Modell (2003) suggests that advances in neuroscience make it possible to view the construction of meaning as a biological property, such as:

> Freud's [A] *Project for a Scientific Psychology* in which emotion and memory form a seamless unified system is seen as an attempt to establish psychoanalysis as a neurobiology of meaning. In the unconscious construction of meaning, metaphor plays a salient role; metaphor is the currency of mind. I have suggested that metaphor functions unconsciously as a pattern detector and thus plays a dominant role in the organizing and categorizing of emotional memory. (p. 255)

To explain this further I will use a scenario of a thirty-five-year-old male client who, in a recent session, was in emotional crisis. It was apparent that this individual needed some *space* to speak without interjection. It was as if he was *crying* uncontrollably and just needed to do so until he felt better and was all *cried out*. He was not crying, though, but speaking. He then stopped speaking and just sat there exhausted. After a few minutes to allow him to compose himself, I asked him how he felt. He said, "A bit bewildered. Actually I feel much better now that all of that's out of me." I then asked, "Where is '*all of that*'?" He right away pointed to the space between where he was sitting and where I was sitting. I asked him if what he was pointing to had a *shape*, to which he answered, after a bit of thought, "Yes" and described the shape. Surprisingly, it was the shape of a person—that of his mother! He went on to say that it is *that* which he has carried with him all his life, and particularly for the last couple of years. In a recent confrontation, this crisis had been triggered. He related to this *pain* and saw himself within it as someone that he did not recognise, and in such a way that it paralysed him in his progress. However, he could not or did not wish to "let it go". He wanted "revenge" but realised now, that somehow by "possessing" this he was "taking his anger out on himself". Not that he wanted to hurt his mother physically, but he wished that he could give this "pain" and emotional paralysis "back to her". This pain that he had given a shape and a name to was something that had controlled him to the point of *emotional paralyses*.

When I asked him how he would release himself from it, he said that he would like to take control of it and to keep it "outside". This "shape" was a "ghost" of his past experiences that he did not wish to be afraid of any longer. He spoke of this "ghost" representing his whole life and all of his experiences. It had influenced and impacted his sense of identity, and his sense of existence—"why" he was alive. He identified with being controlled by his mother and he "did not even live with her or see her that often". He was so consumed by his anger that he did not realise that he was living in a past space—where he was still a little child who was dependent on his mother, to the point where he felt that he could not fend for himself and, therefore would have to die. In other words, to avenge himself, he had even contemplated suicide. This enraged him further to think that he was out of control and powerless to protect himself.

However, he stated that he did not wish to die as he felt that that would be giving in to this "ghost" and his fear of it. He wished to move beyond this "space" where he felt "stuck in time".

It is clear that the above discussion had a metaphorical dimension and is charged with emotional suffering and being in pain. He considered himself a victim of his pain and yet he seemed to hold on to it, the "ghost", which seemed to give him this sense of excitement, and control over his *castrated* self. The metaphor of the "ghost" is the "currency of the mind" accessing emotional memory, which symbolised his desire and in turn, caused a state of pain. He hung on to his pain as if it was a force that overpowered him, yet gave him a sense of a unity within his emotional self.

Melzack (2006) speaks about the brain's objective in maintaining the body/self unity. He visualised:

> the neuromatrix as an assembly whose connections are primarily determined not by experience but by the genes. The matrix, though, could later be sculpted by experience, which would add or delete, strengthen or weaken existing synapses. This processing would also enable the matrix to store the memory of a pain and might thus, account for the frequent reappearance of the same pain. (p. 55)

The matrix is "prewired" with the "whole self" unity as evidenced by Melzack's research of people born without limbs who experienced phantom limbs. In comparison with the concept of Melzack's (2006) neuromatrix, I propose that the "assembly of connections" of the psychomatrix is also genetically prewired and continues to be modulated by experiences.

Historically, according to Freud, whose opinion was echoed by Rank, "the affect of anxiety is a consequence of the event of birth and a repetition of the situation then experienced" (1926, p. 161). Rank went on to propose:

> [I]t would seem that the primal anxiety-affect at birth, which remains operative through life, right up to the final separation from the outer world (gradually becoming a second mother) at death, is from the very beginning not merely an expression of the new-born child's physiological injuries (dyspnoea-constriction-anxiety), but in consequence of the change from a highly pleasurable situation to an extremely painful one, immediately acquires a "psychical" quality of feeling. This *experienced* anxiety is thus the first content of perception, the first psychical act, so to say, to set up barriers; and in these we must recognise the primal repression against the already powerful tendency to re-establish the pleasurable situation just left. (1993, p. 187)

I suggest that the dichotomy of the foetal space, being a space of conflict (pain) as well as a space of comfort (pleasure), continues into the development of the individual—for example, the mother's presence is a source of comfort as well as the source of conflict. This conflict, it seems, continues beyond the birthing event and experience at the end of which the baby is "cut away" and separated from its mother. The trauma and anxieties of loss, fear of rejection, annihilation and loss of control and power over one's own life—fear of the known and the unknown—continue throughout the subject's developmental stages and beyond. The debate on whether or not a foetus can experience pain, at any level and, if it does, at what stage of gestation, is ongoing and will not be discussed in this book. Suffice it to say that if there is a possibility of a foetus experiencing pain—physical and or emotional—within any dimension of its existence, there is a possibility of this experience impacting on the psychosignature as well as the neurosignature of pain, identity, and existence—which is created within the prewired matrices.

This scenario, I believe, can also be perceived as a metaphor for life that the individual is born into the struggle to survive in general, the striving for independence in cutting/breaking away from the dependence of mother, family, or even one's own attitude. It appears to be the same dichotomy of the life instinct and the death instinct, as discussed by Freud (1920g)—the *pain and pleasure* of striving for self-preservation, and gratification, and the striving toward the goal, where there is no longer a desire to strive for self-preservation and gratification, as all desire is fulfilled within the final equilibrium of reaching the place where it all began—death.

Before the end though, and as the subject travels through his developmental phases the phantom of loss already experienced, consciously as well as unconsciously, takes definition and influences thoughts, emotions, and behaviour—from attachment as an infant to attachment as an adult. Holmes (2010) explains his perspective on Bowlby's attachment theory in that the bond between mother and child is a psychological bond in its own right and agrees with Bowlby (1973) who has opined that this bond "provides a language" within which to express the consciousness and existence of this state. Attachment is a "primary motivational system" with its own workings and interface with other motivational systems (p. 63).

The human infant, I propose, is born with an innate sense of desire for attachment. Modell (2003) postulates that the infant is born with the capacity to create attachments: "[T]he human infant is innately predisposed to find meaning in touch, proprioception, and pre-eminently in the affective responsiveness of its caregivers" (p. 556).

Consequently, I assume that the human infant, having been exposed to such experiences, when attached to the mother, is predisposed, undoubtedly, to _re-finding_ the _object_, as a _separated_ entity, through the senses such as touch. He has a body/self image imprinted within his neuromatrix where the imprint is created as the neurosignature unique to that particular individual. Parallel to this neurological system is the emotional and psychological system of the psychomatrix within which is created a particular psychosignature. The imprint of the initial attachment is within this matrix as is the imprint of the initial separation from the mother. The _phantom_ of the psychological and emotional state of being which was once a secure whole self continues to exist in the psychomatrix, hence making the subject predisposed to the state of _being in pain_ due to loss of that, and the desire to satisfy that loss of the once attached object which was part of the body/mind/self unity or whole.

I propose that the sense of _being in pain_ or suffering is a synthesis of the mind/self processes, which modulate the psychosignature (of pain) created within the psychomatrix. Freud stated:

> the remarkable fact that, when there is a psychical diversion brought about by some other interest, even the most intense physical pains fail to arise [...] can be accounted for by there being a concentration of cathexis on the psychical representative of the part of the body which is giving pain. I think it is here that we shall find the point of analogy which has made it possible to carry sensations of pain over to the mental sphere. For the intense cathexis of longing which is concentrated on the missed or lost object [...] creates the same economic conditions as are created by the cathexis of pain which is concentrated on the injured part of the body. (1926d, p. 171)

Here, in _Inhibitions, Symptoms and Anxiety_ (1926d), he examines evidence that there are parallel mechanisms present, physical pain and psychological pain, that lead to emotional suffering, however that the two are destined to interact in order to differentiate the experiential states of _having pain_ and that of _being in pain_ or suffering. Earlier in this same text, he states:

> the line of development which connects this first danger-situation and determinant of anxiety with all the later ones, and we have seen that they all retain a common quality in so far as they signify

in a certain sense a separation from the mother—at first only in a biological sense, next as a direct loss of object and later as a loss of object incurred indirectly. (p. 151)

Freud, as we have already discussed, began to make the connection, between the neurological systems of the body and psychological systems of the mind in *A Project for a Scientific Psychology* (1950a). Since science has progressed to prove this connection, the significance of his research remains as a foundation to study the phantom (experience/ pain) syndrome. The subject gives the phantom, a companion for life, substance according to his own experiences. It is, as research has seen, the "primary motivational system" with its own workings and interface with other motivational systems (Bowlby, 1973).

The phantom limb syndrome

I will continue to explore the phantom limb syndrome, in this chapter, as a metaphor for psychological and emotional pain, a sense of *being in pain* which is present in the subject's life, even though there is no evidence of an immediate, acute trauma or stimulus. I will discuss further the possibility of a psychomatrix similar to the neuromatrix as well as the duality of consciousness pertaining to the sense of *being in pain*.

The phantom limb syndrome is the experience of sensations of pain in a limb or other part of the body, or the sense of a presence of these that do not, or no longer, exist. This is generally reported by amputees as (a) sensations that are not painful—perceptions such as that of movement and the sensation from external stimuli such as touch, pressure, and itching; and (b) as sensations that are painful, such as the perception of burning, tingling, or shooting pains.

An article by Ramachandran and Hirstein (1998) explores the perception of phantom limbs. They suggest that the sensation of the phantom can be triggered by "map expansion neuroplasticity" in which the local brain region that once specialised in controlling the function of the amputated limb, and which is reflected as a discrete "map" in the cerebral cortex of the brain, is taken over by an adjacent brain map such as the face map, thereby expanding the face map. The acquisition of a part of the unused phantom map by the face map results in the perception of sensation in the amputated limb when the face is touched (pp. 1603–1630).

Further research has evidenced that the phantom limb syndrome is not only found in persons whose limbs or other body parts have been amputated, but are also seen in a small percentage of patients with congenitally missing arms or legs. This suggests that at least the basic imprint or map for one's body may be innately specified. The phenomenon provides a valuable opportunity to investigate how nature and nurture interact in the construction of body image by the brain. A patient with leprosy whose hand gets whittled away gradually with progressive sensory loss does *not* have a phantom hand. But if the stump is then amputated, what emerges is not a phantom stump but a whole phantom hand. It is as though the original image of the hand had survived but was inhibited by the stump, only to be resurrected when the stump is amputated (ibid.).

Historical significance

The phenomenon of the phantom limb has been a subject of fascination, but also of ambiguity, awe, and fear, since limblessness has been an inevitable consequence of certain diseases, accidents, genetic disorders, and human activity such as war, violence, and torture, which, as we know, have always been part of society. It is a subject that was neglected and, perhaps, pushed to the realm of the uncanny until about the sixteenth century. There are accounts of the French military surgeon Ambroise Paré in the sixteenth century who was said to be the first to document his observations of this phenomenon. He was aware of phantom limb pain when he wrote in 1551 about the patients who suffered extreme pain in the leg that was no longer present, many months after it had been cut away. These patients imagined that they still had their entire limb. There are accounts written by Descartes where he described phantom sensations in several of his writings, both private and public. One was a letter written to Fromondus on 3 October 1637. Fromondus had been critical of a passage in Descartes' *Optics*, and Descartes now responded to the criticism. His specific purpose was to argue against a "faculty of feeling in the skin or [nerve] membranes"; he believed that sensation must involve the machinery of the brain. Central to his thinking was his belief that perception, which, unlike simple sensation, involves consciousness and understanding, is a distinctly human attribute. It requires the interaction of the immaterial soul with the material brain, which receives basic sensory information from the nerves (Finger & Hustwit, 2003, p. 677).

William Porterfield, a prominent Scottish physician who lived from 1696 to 1771, was possibly the first physician to write about his own experiences after having a leg amputated. He described and interpreted the feelings in his own missing leg. He considered that sensations projected to the missing leg were no more remarkable than colours projected to external objects. For example, Doyle explains, including a quote from Porterfield's diary:

> All things perceived must therefore be present with the mind and in the sensorium where the mind resides … the sense of feeling is diffused thro' all the body. Nay, in some cases it behived to be extended beyond the body itself as in the case of amputations … Having had this misfortune myself, I can the better vouch for the truth of this fact from my own experience, for I sometimes still feel pains and itchings, as if in my tows, heel or ancle and tho it be several years since my leg was taken off.

Before then, most papers had relied on second- or third-hand reports. Not surprisingly:

> Porterfield saw similarities between the visual sensation and that experienced after amputation. He graphically described the sensations of pain and itching, but for some reason did not refer to the papers and reports of others, including Déscartes who, so eloquently, described the suffering of a girl after a limb amputation. (Doyle, 2010)

Phantom limb pain is described in Herman Melville's novel *Moby Dick*, which was first published in 1851. Captain Ahab, who had lost his leg in a skirmish with the great white whale, stated: "A dismasted man never entirely loses the feeling of his old spar [...]. And I still feel the smart of my crushed leg, though it be now so long dissolved." The classical description of phantom limb pain, the most detailed available in the English language is that by Weir Mitchell in 1871. He used the term "sensory hallucinations" to characterise this phenomenon. There are also other examples such as found in the short story *The Case of George*

Dedlow in 1866 (Nathanson, 1988). It is a tale of a young soldier who had undergone surgery due to an injury received in battle. He was unaware when he awoke that his legs had been amputated. He was experiencing cramps in his "legs" and asked an orderly to massage them to relieve the cramping! As mentioned above, Silas Weir Mitchell, in 1871, described the first post-surgical "ghost" occurring in an amputee. He was the first to use the expression "phantom limb". He reported that phantom limb pains, after a traumatic amputation, such as caused by an accident or disaster, were often the same as the pain at the time of the trauma (Ramachandran & Blakeslee, 1998; Melzack & Wall, 1996).

This, I propose, is akin to a psychological trauma. The initial traumatic loss of something or someone significant tends to remain in the emotional system at a similar level of intensity, long after the actual event. Even if the details are not remembered, the pain is.

The phantom limb has been as elusive as pain itself. To explain the mysteries of the existence of pain, people through the ages have been known to resort to a variety of belief systems such as religion and folklore.

According to Halligan (2002), Price and Twombly (1978) came across references to folklore accounts while reviewing the historical literature on phantom limbs, describing the loss and miraculous restoration of body parts, stating that these descriptions were "present in folklore of all kinds the world over, from ancient to modern times", but importantly comprised the central theme of many documented miracle accounts extending back to the tenth century.

During the initial stages of the research, Price became aware that the body parts most often considered were those commonly found to be associated with phantom phenomena (limbs, lip, tongue, nose, eye, penis, breast and nipple, teeth, and viscera). Sensing the possibility that some of these miracle accounts were metaphorical or symbolic allusions to phantom limb phenomena, Price and Twombly (1978) commenced a detailed and critical review of seventy-five historical descriptions. Accounts where the details were indicative of known phantom limb phenomena and where their inclusion in the story did not fulfil any obvious logical or narrative function were considered illustrations of this medical-historical hypothesis.

> Most of these were of the lower limb, and a common miracle involved the leg transplantation by Saint Cosmas and Saint

Damian [...] which dates from the 15th century. Explaining the phenomenological experience of a phantom limb as the product of a miraculous limb restoration therefore represented a metaphorical way that was congruent with religious belief and avoided a direct challenge to folk conceptions of how it was possible to feel a body part that was no longer present. This review enabled Price and Twombly to push back the recorded history of phantom limb phenomena as far back as the 10th century. (p. 256)

Throughout history, there have been many attempts to explain the presence of the ghost of a formerly *alive* limb or part of the body. In ignoring the presence of this phenomenon, as something that could be explored to explain certain mind, body, and self issues, researchers almost missed a significant piece of the puzzle. It goes beyond the mind/body puzzle and reaches the mind/self experiences of the *being in pain* conundrum. Psychological and emotional pain or suffering seems to be the constant in any given individual's life. As pointed out by Ramachandran and Hirstein (1998):

Although patients with this syndrome have been studied extensively since the turn of the century, there has been a tendency among physicians to regard them as enigmatic, clinical curiosities. This neglect of a striking and potentially informative condition is all the more surprising given that research over the past decade has shown that phantom limbs can provide fundamental insights into the functional organisation of the normal human brain and [...] serve as perceptual markers for tracking neural plasticity in the adult brain. (p. 252)

People throughout the ages have also looked to religion and folkloric traditions to explain the existence of pain and suffering in general. In my experience with patients and clients who are suffering with psychological and emotional pain, I see their desire for an escape from their pain, whether it means believing that it is an "act of God" (for the good of something, the pain to gain pleasure/recompense) or the devil (there is evil afoot, guilt and punishment/penance). It seems too painful to look at the state of one's own existence and to know that the control really lives inside oneself, as does one's pain. Hence, here again we see the emotive subject-pain relational entity and that no matter the explanation for the existence of pain there is always a desire to hold it in awe. Emotional pain continues to be placed within the realm of the uncanny where it has the power to provoke excitement and a desire for the other—pain and pleasure beyond or within the pain.

The phantom limb: a metaphor

Why does psychological pain continue to exist in the subject's emotional system, so much so that a past experience is triggered by some stimulus in the present? For example, an altercation at work where one has not been able to express one's concerns or distress about being bullied, and experiences a sense of being rejected, isolated, degraded, and devalued. There is also a physiological reaction such as increased heart rate and perspiration and/or physical weakness or pains in certain parts of the body, such as legs, stomach, and back, and feelings of anxiety, fear, and panic. This scenario may evidence past traumatic experiences of a similar circumstance. The "phantom" of that past event is triggered by this present situation. As Freud postulated:

> A humiliation that was experienced thirty years ago acts exactly like a fresh one throughout the thirty years, as soon as it has obtained access to the unconscious sources of emotion. As soon as the memory of it is touched, it springs into life again and shows itself cathected with excitation which finds a motor discharge in an attack. (1900a, p. 578)

To explain "plasticity" in the unconscious, emotional system of the mind, as discussed in neuroscience, regarding certain phenomena involved in the phantom limb syndrome, it would be valuable to examine Freud's (1899) theory on "screen memories". In the process of repression, a significant (traumatic) memory is suppressed while a less important memory is created to protect the subject from the original memory. I propose that the *space* that is left in the process of the repression is filled by the screen memory. This would act, in my opinion, as the phantom of the original memory.

Freud stated, "instead of the mnemic image which would have been justified by the original event, another is produced which has been to some degree associatively *displaced* from the former one". He further explained that the substituted memory would lack the "important elements" of the original memory. He also said: "It is a case of displacement on to something associated by continuity; or, looking at the process as a whole, a case of repression accompanied by the substitution of something in the neighbourhood (whether in space or time)" (1899, pp. 307–308).

A screen memory is a compromise between repressed elements and the defence against them. Like forgetting important facts that are not retained but, instead, the psychological or psychic significance is displaced onto something that is closely allied or connected, but with less important details. Displacement is the key mechanism at work in screen memories. Freud compared screen memories and dreams. He expressed that because both had visual representations to the subject it was possible that they contained mnemic traces albeit in the form of "dream-thoughts". An analysis of dreams and screen memories allows access to the reality of the true picture of the experiences of the past. He stated that they retained "all of what is essential [...]. They represent the forgotten years of childhood as adequately as the manifest content of a dream represents the dream-thoughts" (1914, p. 148).

What is further relevant to this book is that in the *Three Essays on the Theory of Sexuality* Freud added a note that drew a parallel between screen memories and the fetish, "that behind the first recollection of the fetish's appearance there lies a submerged and forgotten phase of sexual development. The fetish, like a "screen-memory", represents this phase and is thus a remnant and precipitate of it" (1920g, p. 154).

The fetishist aspect of screen memories as with mnemic symbols and images that have been censored, clearly presage Freud's later perspective of fetishism. If a screen memory can be fetishist then can *pain* not fulfil the same desire? This is a question which will be examined subsequently.

Consequently, when these memories, just as other memories, are triggered by an event or experience in the present and bring the original painful experience flooding back it is like the pain of the phantom limb. The pain of the phantom is the same intensity, then, as the original experience of pain in the physical realm as in the psychical realm. There is *something* that exists even though it does not. However, the pain of the phantom is the same intensity—but there is no limb! Is pain the phantom or is it the (missing) limb? There is a sense of a limb—as there is a sense of an event or experience (in the past)—a conscious awareness of what has been buried in the unconscious.

I propose that in this case the subject's relationship with (phantom) pain is a type of defence mechanism to ward of the memory of a past traumatic or tragic event. Fetishist in nature, pain fulfils the aspect of disavowal, of possessing that which is lost and the pleasure inherent within that pain. This element of disavowal is to be found in psychoanalytic theory. Freud identifies this as a defence mechanism where "the subject" refuses "to recognise the reality of a traumatic perception". He relates this to the "castration complex" where the "traumatic perception" occurs at the first sight of the female genitalia. Children disavow the absence of a penis and believe that they do see one all the same (Evans, 2006 p. 43).

In Lacan's account, the realisation that the cause of desire is always a lack is that which disavowal concerns. "Disavowal is the failure to accept that lack which causes desire and the belief that desire is caused by a presence (e.g. the fetish)" (Evans, 2006, p. 44).

The neuromatrix theory is that (physical/neurological) pain is caused as the *brain* attempts to maintain the fidelity of the body/self unity. Similarly, the psychomatrix theory is that (emotional/psychological) pain is caused as the mind attempts to maintain the integrity of the *self* without the lack, when in fact there is a lack—desire for the lost object and the desire of the other.

The phantom limb syndrome is the sensation that a limb persists despite its having been amputated. Whilst extremely common—sixty to eighty per cent of amputees report the experience—it is often felt as extremely painful. One of the interesting things to note when we think about this syndrome using the theory of the mirror stage is that one of the most effective treatments for this pain involves the therapeutic use of mirrors. Apart from it referring to a libidinal relationship with the body image, an element of Lacan's mirror stage theory is its referral to a dual relationship between the ego and the body, however it also refers to a link between the imaginary and the real. The visual identity which is given from the mirror provides an imaginary "whole" to the experience of a fragmented real. The mirror stage describes the formation of the ego via the process of identification. In this case, the ego is the result of identifying with one's own specular image (Lacan, 1992, 2006).

Keeping this in mind, we may be able to understand the emotional effect of the so-called mirror box experiment created by Ramachandran. This was and still is a treatment that involves a patient inserting both his good and "phantom" limb into a box divided into two, the sections separated by a mirror (Ramachandran & Blakeslee, 1998). When the patient moves his good limb, he sees in the mirror next to it the reflected image of a symmetrical limb in the place where he feels his phantom limb. By this method the patient is able to alleviate the feelings reported by many sufferers—that their phantom limb is clenched or contorted in a painful position.

> From a Lacanian perspective we might wonder whether this kind of visual-kinaesthetic feedback is not replicating exactly the kind of motor mastery over the "fragmented" body, the *corps morcelé*, that Lacan describes as the experience of the infant prior to the mirror stage? (Lacan, 2003)

The article goes on to suggest that indeed, Lacan makes a reference to phantom limb syndrome in *Some Reflections on the Ego* in 1950:

> The meaning of the phenomenon called "phantom limb" is still far from being exhausted. The aspect which seems to me especially worthy of notice is that such experiences are essentially related to the continuation of a pain which can no longer be explained by local irritation; it is as if one caught a glimpse here of the existential relation of a man with his body-image in this relationship with such a narcissistic object as the lack of a limb ... ["phantom limb" syndrome] leads us to suspect that the cerebral cortex functions like a mirror, and that it is the site where the images are integrated in the libidinal relationship which is hinted at in the theory of narcissism. (Lacan, 2003, p. 298)

For the purposes of my book, this is a valid perspective of the phantom limb syndrome. The "mirror box" experiment proved useful in eliminating, for the most part, the pain or cramping or paralysis of the phantom limb. The brain (optics) and body as well as the mind interaction is clear, as he evidences that a "learned paralysis can be unlearned" by engaging the phantom and fulfilling the desire of the brain processes—for the arm to "move". This is done by sending a visual message to the phantom arm to a reflection of the existing arm. The phantom arm is "hidden" behind a mirror that is actually reflecting the existing arm on the opposite side. The reflection makes it appear as if the phantom arm exists and is real. The visual message is sent to the reflection tricking the brain into believing that this was, actually, the missing arm. The existing arm is moved making it appear that the phantom is moving therefore, making the brain assume that the phantom arm that was "paralysed" is now able to move. The neuromatrix theory holds its value as the substrate of the whole body is kept "intact" by bringing meaning to the image in the mirror—a metaphor with emotional connotations that has implications for the possibility of a *psychomatrix*.

Pain is temporarily relieved when desire is satisfied, but returns once more as this diminishes and brings a renewed desire (Schopenhauer, 1969, pp. 318–319). I assume then, that the phantom of the real object of desire can never be eliminated as the presence of the phantom limb can never be eliminated as long as the desire for the real (object) limb remains.

The relationship of the subject and his body then, speaks of the subject's relationship with his pain. It is a narcissistic desire for that which is lost in order to be "complete" knowing that this is an impossibility. This very knowledge, which is painful, is in itself a pleasure as excitement of the search continues to fill the void that has been created by loss.

Duality of consciousness

According to Freud, the conscious mind is everything that we are aware of and the mental processes of thinking and expressing oneself in rational language. Consciousness, he explained, is a "particular function" of the mental processes. At that time he explained that when the conscious system becomes aware of an experience there is no imprint left on its system: "Thus we should be able to say that the excitatory process becomes conscious in the systems Cs. but leaves no permanent trace behind there." However, the imprint is actually left on the adjacent system (of the unconscious) (1920g, p. 25). The key element is the "excitatory process". It seems that there are other elements at work that cause emotional experiences to be tucked away in the unconscious.

Referring back to his work in the *Project* (1950a) Freud explains that consciousness is not the only system that leaves traces or imprints behind. He discusses further that this is the process by which memory (and motive) is created. Stimulus from external and internal environments cause "excitations" in the other systems of the individual not just in the conscious system, which impact memory and leave behind traces and imprints. He stated that the memory traces left behind thus "have nothing to do with the fact of becoming conscious; indeed they are often most powerful and most enduring when the process which left them behind was one which never entered consciousness" (1920g, pp. 24–26).

More recent studies are not far off from Freud's hypotheses, as consciousness is understood in many different ways such as the state of being awake, of being aware of oneself or one's surroundings, being able to focus our attention or to make voluntary decisions. It is a "highly subjective quality of experience" (Chalmers, 1997). The question of duality comes into view as we consider our previous discussion about the experience of pain, physical and psychological—*having pain* and *being in pain*. It seems that this would bring into perspective the notion of duality. According to Chalmers, the problem of consciousness begs a discussion and focuses in on the concepts of the mind. Mainly there are two concepts of mind: phenomenological, "conscious experience", and psychological, "causal or explanatory basis for behaviour". At the heart of consciousness lies the concept of experience. Chalmers says, "we can say that a mental state is conscious if it has a *qualitative feel*—an associated quality of experience. These qualitative feelings are also known as phenomenal qualities or *qualia* for short" (1997, pp. 3–4).

There are, according to this research, several types of conscious experiences, among them being the experience of pain, other bodily sensations, conscious thought, emotions, and the sense of self. The experience of pain is most prominent of experiences as it is distinct from all other experience and can include sensory experiences from "fierce burns" to "sharp pricks to dull aches". Pain can also be allied to sensations of "hunger pangs, itches" and "tickles". There are other types of bodily sensations such as experiences associated with "orgasm, or the feeling of hitting one's funny bone". Emotions can include the experiences of happiness or sadness and depression and anger and pleasure that encompass our experiences. The more cognitive aspects of emotions are those that involve anxiety, pent-up tension, and a sudden release of pleasure (ibid., p. 9).

Of the experience of the sense of self, Chalmers states:

> [O]ne sometimes feels that there is something to conscious experience that transcends all these specific elements: a kind of background hum, for instance, that is somehow fundamental to

consciousness and that is there even when the other components are not. This phenomenology of self is so deep and intangible that it sometimes seems illusory, consisting in nothing over and above specific elements such as those listed above. Still, there seems to be something to the phenomenology of self, even if it is very hard to pin down. (1997, p. 10)

The concept of consciousness, as well as the unconscious, is significant to the phantom limb scenario as we consider it as a metaphor for the self/mind unity and the subject-pain relationship. The subject is conscious of his pain be it physical or psychological, within the duality of phenomenological and psychological dimensions of his existence. As Chalmers states above, "the phenomenology of self is so deep and intangible that it sometimes seems illusory" (ibid.), pain brings to consciousness an orchestration of sensations that do not always "sound" harmonious to the unities of body, brain and mind. However, within all of that there is the "background hum" of the experience of the self and its relationship with pain. The subject is conscious of his *relationship* as a "hum" that tells him that he exists. Not always in the sphere of the conscious, indeed it is mostly unconscious, and as Freud (1923b) has said, what is conscious is only the tip of the iceberg.

Part of the conscious mind includes our memory which is not always part of consciousness, but can be retrieved easily at any time and brought into our awareness. Freud called this ordinary memory the preconscious. In contrast, the unconscious is a collection of experiences and of feelings, thoughts, urges, and memories that are present outside of our conscious awareness. Within the unconscious lie the representations of memories that are mostly feelings of pain, anxiety, and conflict that are unacceptable or unpleasant. According to Freud, the unconscious consists of all that is repressed and continues to influence our behaviour and experience, even though we are unaware of these underlying influences. My question here is that if the unconscious holds what is repressed, feelings of pain, anxiety and conflict that are unacceptable or unpleasant, is it not feasible that this is the seat of the psychomatrix within which is created the psychosignature of *pain*?

Freud proposed:

[W]e have arrived at the term or concept of the unconscious along another path, by considering certain experiences in which mental *dynamics* play a part. We have found—that is, we have been obliged to assume—that very powerful mental processes or ideas exist (and here a quantitative or economic factor comes into question for the first time) which can produce all the effects in mental life that ordinary ideas do (including effects that can in their turn become conscious as ideas), though they themselves do not become conscious. (1923b, p. 14)

The mental processes that Freud speaks of above, I would argue, are what essentially create the psychosignature of pain. I propose that pain is the "economic factor" in consciousness however pain is also the qualitative aspect of consciousness.

Freud (1916–1917) explains that there are two different kinds of unconscious. He said that although what is repressed is unconscious, it is not so simple as to say that the unconscious is all that is repressed: He states, "the repressed is part of the unconscious" (p. 166).

The unconscious comprises, on the one hand, acts which are merely latent, temporarily unconscious, but which differ in no other respect from conscious ones and, on the other hand, processes such as repressed ones, which if they were to become conscious would be bound to stand out in the crudest contrast to the rest of the conscious processes. (ibid., p. 172)

The unconscious holds representations of our every experience, some of those that are repressed manifest in various forms of behaviour and others do not. Albeit there are experiences that are negative, there are also those that are positive. What is negative, though, it appears, tends to impact the conscious state, and what is significant is that the impact on the unconscious, from all experiences, is undoubtedly imprinted on many levels. Take for example, the process of repression and the many mechanisms to maintain it—such as denial—and its ensuing manifestations within the anxieties. And when we consider the profundity of pain and its capacity to permeate every aspect of human existence we can only begin to gauge the power (and need) of its existence, especially when we consider that another dimension of pain is pleasure. In his explanation of the theory of the "pleasure principle" in *Beyond the Pleasure Principle*, Freud (1920g) stated that whatever has been repressed will find its way out or manifest itself in one way or another. He speaks of the compulsion to repeat as one such manifestation. An experience that was unacceptable to the consciousness of the subject is repressed in his unconscious, however in seeking an outlet for expression it shows itself in repetitive behaviour, demanding to be heeded. Freud explained as well that it is not the unconscious that is resisting the exposition of what is within. The resistance, he states, "arises from the same higher strata and systems of the mind which originally carried out repression" (ibid., p. 19).

This brings to mind a mechanism that is akin to Melzack and Wall's theory of the "gate control system" within the central nervous system. There are certain neuronal cells that allow the gate to *open* to allow certain stimuli in, while other cells act to close the gate to prevent other stimuli to enter thus controlling the level and quality of pain. The many domains of the individual's environment, inevitably, impact on their tolerance level. The emotive aspect of pain is, I argue, imprinted in the parallel system of the psychomatrix within the unconscious becoming part of the conglomerate. Within the systems of the unconscious a similar activity implicating the ego, allow or prevent certain ideas into the conscious manifesting in certain behaviours. The repetitive quality of these behaviours is thus influenced.

Freud discusses the evidence in the act of repetition of a behaviour or thought in order to gain pleasure as in the child's play of hide and seek or of the appearance and disappearance of a "wooden spool via a piece of string". We have the ability to allow or disallow a painful event into the realm of our reality via our desire to find pleasure from the pain of loss—which is like a "piece of string" that we have a hold on. Adults indulge in similar behaviours that can also manifest within the process of therapy. Once something is brought to the forefront or into conscious awareness it needs to be worked through in order to alleviate the trauma attached to it. Freud points out: "[T]his is convincing proof that, even under the dominance of the pleasure principle, there are ways and means enough of making what is in itself unpleasurable into a subject to be recollected and worked over in the mind" (1920g, p. 17).

The unconscious systems of the mind, I have proposed, are the seat of the psychomatrix and where the psychosignature of pain is innately created and modulated by experiences. The experience of *being in pain* is the "phantom" of the collection of repressed experiences that impact the subject's existence and identity. Pain, unlike pleasure, is an entity that remains within the subject's emotional make-up, within the unconscious, in one aspect or another. This pain has a powerful and dramatic effect on, not only, the body/self (somatic dimension) unity but also, and especially, the subject/object (psychic/emotional dimension) relationship. The phantom of pain remains as a phenomenal experience in the subject's consciousness—like a "hum" in the background it is there, like a companion, in every thought and behaviour (Chalmers, 1997).

Since Hoffman's (1954) review on the literature on the phantom limb syndrome there have been advancements in science to facilitate further understanding of this phenomenon For example, Melzack's (1993) neuromatrix theory. However, in this article he adds an important psychological and psychoanalytical perspective:

> The pattern of body image consists of processes which construct and build up with the help of sensations and perceptions, but the emotional processes are the force and the source of energy of these constructive processes, and they direct them. [...] The phantom of an amputated person is, therefore, the reactivation of a given perceptive pattern by emotional forces. (ibid., p. 264)

How the subject reacts to loss of his limb is contingent upon how they perceive their own body, or body image. The subject's perception of his body or their "self-evaluation" is influenced by their environment. Therefore, it is possible that "'the psychical origin' of pain may be projected into some peripheral area. One's position or status, so to speak, in life is in a good share dependent on his self-evaluation in and on his environment" (ibid.).

Hoffman (1954) suggested:

> [T]he phantom limb represents a narcissistic inability to renounce the integrity of the body or acknowledge the symbolic castration and thereby accept a relatively inferior position and/or separation from the world. [...] The final picture of a phantom is, to a great extent, dependent on the emotional factors in the life situation. The phantom is a model of how psychic life in general is going on. The interaction (between the periphery and the centre) is based upon the playful multiplication of psychic experiences. [...] The body and each portion has connected with it some emotional significance derived from early familial conditioning and of the later cultural values. (ibid., p. 265)

I propose that loss of a limb or body part brings to the forefront the reality of object-loss and the traumatic reminder of the threat of castration. The depth and complexity of loss disallows one to fill the emptiness with anything other than what is lost, hence, the "phantom", which is a representation of that which is lost.

As Freud had evidenced throughout his clinical work at the turn of the nineteenth century, so it is still true. Regardless of the plethora of research in the field of psychology, it has been established that our thoughts, feelings and consequent behaviour are motivated (and inspired) by our brain's (neurological) and our mind's (psychological and emotional) ability to store memories. However, it is not just the storing of memories, but the censorship of what is stored that is significant. Freud postulated that in the unconscious is stored the representations of our experiences. The very statement that there are "representations" is clear—most things that we remember are not exact details of the actual events. It may feel as if it is the exact same experience as it happened in the past; however, it is our mind's desire to maintain an integrity of the experience. This is the "phantom" that remains with us. A phantom of the real event, however it has no substance except what we individually allow it to have. What substance we allow it to have is contingent upon our innate psychomatrix and the signature that is created within it. The psychosignature that is particular to the individual's *being in pain* or *suffering*.

Modell's (2003, p. 556) statement that "as the emotional interchanges that occur between infants and their caretakers are repetitive, these repetitions form recognisable patterns of feeling states that are invariably backed by memory and will serve later as templates of relatedness", is an example of the creation of the psychosignature. This is the state of being that the subject finds himself in and this is what he needs to contend with.

The phantom pain is a conscious experience, with neurological explanations however, the quality of the pain springs from unconscious wishes and fantasies which seem to fill the lack and desire for the lost object—an effort to save the *self* from a disintegration of the whole.

Pain as an object

A trauma or tragic experience is a breach in the emotional systems of the mind and adds to the sense of loss which throws the subject into a state of *suffering* or *being in pain* which consequently initiates a mourning state. This however, has the potential to develop into the state of depression or as Freud (1917) termed it, "melancholia".

In observing patients who are in therapy, I am curious to know why they do not want to "know" their suffering or pain. Or maybe they know and are rejecting it so as to prolong their state of *having pain*—but why? To have pain is to know something about the external "torturer"— pain that is being inflicted in contrast to being in pain or suffering is to know something of the "internal torturer". The concern here is with this "internal torturer". In either case there is an element of pain being inflicted, pain used as an instrument or a thing—a perverse manifestation. As Abel-Hirsch (2006) states:

> "[T]he differentiation of pain as a felt thing that is used and pain that is suffered and thence discovered by the person is consistent with the parallel development of thought on perversion that looks at the way disavowal or misrepresentation of reality can both be regarded as constructions rather than discoveries." (p. 101)

I propose that the subject's relationship with pain is seen within his perception of the reality of pain within his perverse relationship to reality. I propose that pain is an object libidinally cathected by the subject. Pain is the object that is within the space carved out by that which was lost. Pain is desire for that which is lost as well as the representation of what is lost. Therefore, seeking fulfilment is to find pleasure within pain. It is an object used to provoke an experience of *having pain*—pain felt as something externally inflicted, or to invoke an internal experience of suffering or *being in pain*.

In examining the phenomenon of phantom pain, we can identify a *something* that fills the lack in the whole—body or the psyche. Pain is what is left within the space where a "breach" has occurred. What exactly is pain, specifically psychological and emotional pain is a question that presents a problem. For in the effort to describe this pain the significance of the experience of pain is lost. We use the analogy of Pontalis' theory of the dream-object within the dream that is likened to a vessel or container. He states that his "hypothesis is that every dream, as an object in the analysis, refers to the maternal body. [...] Dreaming is above all the attempt to maintain an impossible union with the mother, to preserve an undivided whole, to move in a space prior to time" (1981, p. 29).

Pain, then, can be constructed as an object to be used upon the body and or the psyche, to have pain or to be in pain. The experience of pain is subjective and so is experienced, first of all in, the narcissistic dimension of the subject. It is the object that fills the desire of the lost object. Abel-Hirsch quotes Britton: "[T]he suffering is felt to arise within the self as a consequence of something missing" (2006, pp. 100–101).

Whether it is physical pain or psychic pain there is a merging of the two states especially in individuals that experience severe circumstances, such as amputations and chronic pain syndromes, or other extreme life events such as war and terrorism, disease or childhood sexual abuse. Moreover, it is the state of *having pain* that transforms to the state of *suffering* or *being in pain* as the experience of an event passes through the psychomatrix and is modulated by the psychosignature. Here suffering becomes the staying entity, the memory, in the (unconscious) mind which, in turn, influences one's state of existence and their sense of identity. The aspects of identity and existence which are impacted by the state of *being in pain*, go back to infantile loss and desire for self-preservation, primary desire to return to a state of pleasure and possession of the object and secondary narcissism—the development of a sense of self, independent of the object yet, retaining some aspects of the primary narcissism.

To examine the theory of pain as an object I would argue here that it is in this objectification that we can identify the formulation of the fetishist object. As stated by Abel-Hirsch: "It is widely recognized that perversion is not limited to a person's sexual behaviour, but may influence all of an individual's experiences, relations, and attitudes to reality" (ibid., p. 99). Therefore, the experience of pain whether it is physical as in *having pain*, or psychological as in *being in pain*, may be constructed and objectified to be used in the perverse sphere of experience.

As Freud discussed in his *Project* (1905a) and carried forward in his subsequent work, pain in the physical system of the body can be imprinted in the parallel systems of the emotional or psychological systems of the mind. Pain thus imprinted is recategorised to that of suffering and the phantom of a previous experience, physical or psychological. However, a differentiation is irrelevant as in either case there is, as Abel-Hirsch suggested, a "parallel development of thought on perversion that looks at the way disavowal or misrepresentation can be used to obscure an unwanted discovery of reality. The misuse of pain and the misrepresentation of reality can both be regarded as constructions" (ibid., p. 101).

The matrix

As discussed earlier in this book, the matrix is defined as "an array of circuit elements ... for performing a specific function as interconnected". This array of neurons in a neuromatrix, Melzack (1993) suggests is genetically programmed. "The neuromatrix distributed throughout many areas of the brain, comprises a widespread network of neurons that generate patterns, process information that flows through them, and ultimately produces the pattern that is felt as a whole body." The patterns vary according to individual subjectivity; however, the neurosignature of the "whole body" remains constant maintaining the sense of a body/self unity (pp. 622–623).

The brain/body/mind relationship exists in order to maintain the integrity of the unity of the "whole". This relationship has a historical significance to survival and self-preservation. As described by Melzack, the neuromatrix is inherent to an individual's make-up and functioning. It is within this matrix that is created, by the impressions of historical experience, cognitive and behavioural responses to day to day events that are essential to functioning. As Melzack stated:

> The output of the body neuromatrix [...] is directed at two systems:
> (1) the neuromatrix that produces awareness of the output, and (2)
> a neuromatrix involved in overt action patterns. In this discussion,
> it is important to keep in mind that just as there is a steady stream
> of awareness (even during the dream episodes of sleep), there is
> also a steady output of behaviour (including movements during
> sleep). (1993, p. 625)

The neurosignature that is created within the neuromatrix is a structure that governs the processes and systems of the body including the body/brain relationship in order to maintain the integrity for this unity. If there is a breach in this integrity, such as loss of a limb, it reacts in such a way to attempt to recreate or reconstruct this unity. In further consideration of this I propose that this system and process of maintaining a whole is a metaphor for the subject's desire: (a) for a union with that which he has lost (the mother) and so overcoming the trauma of loss, to belong, and to overcome the fear of annihilation; and (b) for seeking pleasure beyond pain. The subject's desire to maintain that which is not possible (pain), in a sense of wholeness (state of pleasure without desire), is what drives his thoughts and behaviours that attempt to bring equilibrium to his existence.

Maintaining the integrity of the mind/self or body/self unity could be at the expense of certain realities—an example of *having pain*, "I know that my leg is not there however, it is there as the pain tells me that it exists" or another example of *being in pain*, a forty year old patient stated, as he had a number of times, throughout his therapy, "*my* father is dead now, but he was a cruel man. I remember his abuse and I hate him now as I did then. I realise that he does not have the power to control my life anymore, but I live in that place, and I still suffer and feel emotionally paralysed. This suffering, in the first place reminds me that I do not wish to be like him." In response to a question he stated that he enjoys being aggressive and "letting ignorant people know how I feel about their stupidity". The phantom of his past experience clearly fills the place of loss in the form of pain that manifests in aggression, and a need for revenge. The further he "runs away" from wanting to be like his father the closer he gets to it.

The emotional state of pain, of *being in pain*, is one that does not "go away" and is a "phantom" of one's past. Just as there is a relationship between the brain and the body/self unity to explain the existence of a phantom limb, there is a relationship between the conscious and the unconscious to explain the existence of the subject-pain relationship.

The phantom limb syndrome was of interest to the research of Melzack (1993) due to his previous studies and his theory of brain functions. The problem that fascinated him was that the absence of a limb, due to amputation or genetic dysfunctions, did not preclude having pain in that "limb". This was a phantom that he wanted to pursue to understand the workings of the brain and the implications of the imprinting of experiences, particularly those of pain. This neurosignature of the body, created within the neuromatrix, responds to any signal that deviates from its body/self image and unity.

The fascination is with the phenomenon of the presence of pain when there is no, acute physical, psychological and emotional, stimuli. Following the physical experience of the sense of *having pain*, the experience of *being in pain*, that of suffering continues in the subject's emotional and psychic dimension. It is the same circumstance when an emotional or psychological trauma has passed. The suffering remains manifesting in behaviour or physical symptoms. The subject-pain relationship, in this case is to satisfy the mourning, loss and ambiguity of what was once or should be or should have been a whole unit. Pain here is the object which fills this void.

It would be the cathexis that the ego cannot execute, therefore remains a perverse feature of the ego's desire—the subject's unconscious, masochistic need to have pain, and to manipulate it, in order to *be in pain* in order to sustain the possibility of regaining what was lost, or creating a fantasy of what it should be. In reading Merleau-Ponty (2002), I came across a statement that adds to the already discussed perspectives:

> [W]hat it is in us which refuses mutilation and disablement is an I committed to a certain physical and inter-human world, who continues to tend toward his world despite handicaps and amputations and who, to this extent, does not recognize them *de jure*. The refusal of the deficiency is only the obverse of our inherence in a world, the implicit negation of what runs counter to the natural momentum which throws us into our tasks, our cares, our situation, our familiar horizons. To have a phantom arm is to remain open to all the actions of which the arm alone is capable: it is to retain the practical field which one enjoyed before mutilation. (p. 94)

I take it one step further to say that besides the desire "to retain the practical field which one enjoyed before mutilation" there is also a desire to obtain that kind of enjoyment or pleasure, the possibility of such a circumstance or to have that which one imagines or thinks one should have. Therefore, "to have a phantom arm is to remain open to all the actions of which the arm alone is capable"—and I suggest that the phantom limb is a metaphor for the phantom of an emotional attachment from the past. It is also a means of avenging that which caused the fear of annihilation. Pain is the phantom of what is locked away in the unconscious—loss of object. It is the object. The motive of the subject's alliance with pain is to cause the (maternal) object pain by his *being in pain*. Pain is then, not only a defence against the loss but also a reminder of that which was lost.

I saw in my patients a dimension of pleasure in their desire to retain the "possibility of possibilities" (Kierkegaard, in Hong & Hong, 2000, pp. 138–139)—the anxiety that gave substance to their relationship to (their) pain meant that the possibility of achieving that which they desired existed. Equally the possibility of the opposite was also present however this anxiety was "worth having" if the former were to materialise.

The theory of the neuromatrix also implicates the psychological dimensions of pain. Melzack (1993) postulates that the brain "generates perceptual experience even when no external inputs occur" (p. 628). As discussed earlier, it is clear when we consider a matrix within the network of the brain function that is in continual and cyclical transmission. According to Melzack's (1993) article on the phantom limb there are three major neural circuits in the brain that are influenced to create the qualities of experiences. These are the:

> sensory pathway passing through the thalamus to the somatosensory cortex. A second system must consist of the pathways leading through the reticular formation of the brain stem to the limbic system, which is critical for emotion and motivation. A final system consists of cortical regions important to recognition of the self and to the evaluation of sensory signals. A major part of this system is the parietal lobe, which in studies of brain-damaged patients has been shown to be essential to the sense of self. (ibid., pp. 54–55)

Suffering or the sense of *being in pain* is retained, in a parallel system, as a reminder of that which is lost and to maintain the possibility of fulfilment. The possibility that there is also created, simultaneously, a psychomatrix within the unconscious from within which a psychosignature, specific to emotional pain, as discussed, becomes increasingly viable.

Melzack (1993) stated that "experience would enable the matrix to store the memory of a pain from a gangrenous ulcer and might thus account for the frequent reappearance of the same pain in phantom limbs" (ibid.). Even though impressions of such an event are stored as impressions on the neuro-circuitry of the brain I suggest that the emotional meaning of this can only be stored in the psychological processes, which would, in turn, confirm the existence and significance of a parallel matrix, in the emotional, unconscious system, which is specific to pain.

Even though the neuromatrix affects the processing of body, brain and psychological functioning, it does not account for the *persistent* presence of psychological and emotional pain. I will argue that here is where the concept of a psychomatrix could play a role. Because *being in pain*, even though connected to having pain, is an independent process.

As such, the neuromatrix and psychomatrix integrate and cooperate to create the unity of function—mind and brain (and body). The emotional and psychological self is, I propose, essential in the development of the subject's identity and sense of existence.

In reading Kierkegaard the essential factor to emotional survival and growth is, what I would name, the *anxiety factor*. It is accepted that there is a dimension of fear within anxiety, however Kierkegaard states that anxiety differs in that it (anxiety) "is freedom's actuality as the possibility of possibility" (Hong & Hong, 2000, p. 139).

He goes on to posit that anxiety has psychological ambivalence: "anxiety is a *sympathetic antipathy* and *an antipathetic sympathy*", and further that it is an essential developmental process. He states: "[T]his anxiety belongs so essentially to the child that he cannot do without it. Though, it captivates him by its pleasing anxiousness [*beaengstelse*]" (ibid.). He relates the example from a Grimm's fairy tale about a young man's curiosity about anxiety that takes him on an adventure of discovery only to prove that "this is an adventure that every human being must go through—to learn to be anxious in order that he may not perish either by never having been in anxiety or by succumbing in anxiety. Whoever has leaned to be anxious in the right way has learned the ultimate" (ibid., p. 153).

From our primal history, this could be one "phantom" that has its use! It could possibly be an explanation for the phenomenological presence of *being in pain* or *suffering*. In treating my clients presenting with a variety of issues I observe that the core of their illness is pain, which is the core factor in anxiety. However, it is where they have "succumbed in anxiety" which is similar to "discovering pain" which Bion (1970) speaks about. My speculation is that this "succumbing in anxiety" is a breach to the emotional and psychological system and circuitry within the psychomatrix. I propose that just as when a limb is amputated the neuromatrix attempts to normalise the body/self image, by continuous transmission of messages in spite of no response from the site of the previously attached limb, so it is when there is a breach in emotional stability, the psychomatrix struggles to maintain the mind/self unity by an increase in feelings of anxiety. However, when the emotional response mechanism is paralyzed due to acute trauma it creates a "phantom" in the form of a behaviour such as, aggression, chronic pain, or addiction or no action at all. The psychosignature continues to modulate inputs from the experience and respond in such a way that the cognitive and behavioural outputs are those of an acute increase in *having pain* that may be perceived as *being in pain* or *suffering*. It is similar to what Ramachandran calls "a learned paralysis" (1998, p. 47).

The sense of *having pain* in a phantom limb then, is really an expression of *being in pain*. There is no real limb to provide the physical sensation of having pain; however, the body/self unity within the neuromatrix continues to relay messages to the missing limb. However, the messages are not only relayed to that part of the limb of the body they also traverse the imprint or the signature within the matrix, hence, the sense of the presence of the limb as it was before amputation. It is an attempt of the brain to maintain the whole body integrity (Ramachandran & Blakesless, 1998). I propose that it is an effort on the part of a relationship that is created between the brain and the body/self unity, as in the case of the relationship between the subject and pain.

I propose that as with the body, when no emotional or psychological stimulus is present, the mind/self system fills the lack, to maintain the "phantom", through manifestations of neurotic symptoms such as anxieties, obsessions and addictions—grounded in desire and loss. The phantom limb syndrome thus remains a metaphor for the experience of *being in pain*.

Further observation, in patients, has evidenced that similar to the phantom limb being felt as a real object (in the brain), emotional and psychological pain is a phantom, in the mind, causing the subject to *be in pain* or *suffer*.

These are the misrepresentations and disavowal that Steiner (1995) discusses and states: "I believe that these misrepresentations are central to our understanding of perversions and that they arise from a quite specific mechanism in which contradictory versions of reality are allowed to exist simultaneously" (p. 90).

Pain has the power to take over the subject's life by becoming the object and creating the distance needed, which allows the subject-pain relationship to function. This objectification allows pain to be that which is desired. Pain becomes the object that fills the loss but it is also a reminder of the loss and the desire to regain that which was lost. As long as pain poses the possibility of pleasure and filling the loss, pain remains the fetish object that is (unconsciously) sought.

The following is a case scenario of phantom limb syndrome. As a metaphor, I hope to apply it to explain my theory of the subject pain relationship and its impact on identity and existence.

The case of Y

I would like to examine the case of Y as it had an array of multifaceted dimensions which were interesting mainly due to her psychotic illness. In many ways, Y's gradual mental deterioration put her into a different "world". Her *reality* was that of being a "slave" and "imprisoned" in a place where she had very few choices. She had, however, reconciled to this reality by setting up defences to protect herself. For example, her refusal to bathe or take medication was her way to keep her "slave masters" at bay. The loss of her leg became part of her enslavement as for her, having the freedom to walk was like having the freedom to "walk away" a sense of freedom that (at that time) she did not have.

When she complained of having pains in the (amputated) leg, or when she felt itchiness in that same leg or on any other part of her body, it was the only time she *experienced* her body. This experience seemed to be the only time she felt "free" of her sense of slavery and felt instead a sense of omnipotence over the reality (her environment), which was influenced by the doctors, nurses and social workers reminding her that she needed to bathe, eat and take medication because of her circumstances—limb loss, pain, diabetes, loss of her daughter etc. This was a time when the "phantom" of her existence was her closest ally, and her means to fulfilling her (self-preservative and sexual) desire.

My theory of the psychomatrix and phantom pain is evidenced in Y's relationship with her pain—the reason for its existence in her life—and how this had impacted on her sense of identity and existence. This case was of interest to my book due to the dual aspects of Y's diagnosis: her psychotic illness as well as her neurotic symptoms. The disavowal mechanism in Y's case harks back to a Freudian perspective where he links it to psychosis as well as fetishism and as Evans (2005) suggests:

> [I]n these clinical conditions, disavowal is always accompanied by the opposite attitude (acceptance of reality), since it is rarely or perhaps never "possible for the ego's detachment from reality to be carried through completely" [Freud, *An Outline of Psycho-Analysis*, S. E., 23, p. 141]. The coexistence in the ego of these two

contradictory attitudes to reality leads to what Freud terms the splitting of the ego. (p. 43)

Historical background

Y was a female in her mid-fifties, of African origin, and generally of good humour. She had travelled to the UK to escape the traumas of war and poverty. After a period of physical and psychological deterioration, and subsequent hospitalisation and treatment, Y was placed in a nursing home for respite care for an extended period of recuperation and further assessment. Ten years earlier Y's twelve-year-old-child had died in a roadside accident. Reports indicated that this event had triggered the late onset of a psychotic breakdown that had progressed into an enduring, persistent, psychotic disorder categorised as schizophrenia. This resulted in her being on antipsychotic medication ever since. Prior to her hospitalisation that brought this case to my attention, Y had lived independently and had a routine that she followed religiously every day. She was well known in her community and had a boyfriend who visited her daily, as she did not want him to live with her. Part of her routine was that she would allow him to bathe her once a week.

While in the nursing home, Y recuperated for a while from the acute illness (disease progression, and surgery due to phantom leg pains). Soon she began to refuse her medications except for medication for the pain in her phantom limb. As time went on, she also began to refuse to wash, bathe, change her clothes and look after her basic hygiene, and eat the food that was served to her in the home.

During *lucid* moments, where she seemed to be engaging, Y would repeatedly and sorrowfully relate the story of how she lost her child and the blame that she placed on herself for not being able to prevent the accident.

The significance of this case is that Y developed many symptoms such as severe, all-over itching, heart problems, weight gain, circulatory problems, depression, type 2 diabetes, and fungal infection in her feet. This resulted in gangrene setting in on one of her legs, below her knee. Failed attempts to slow the gangrene resulted in a below the knee amputation to stop the spread of further infection and deterioration. At the time of my contact with Y, she was presenting psychotic symptoms as well as neurotic tendencies.

Presenting symptoms

Y was clinically diagnosed with schizophrenia, *a psychotic disorder*, in her thirties. There were positive symptoms such as delusions as well as negative symptom such as a degree of poverty of speech and of thought content, anhedonia (the absence of pleasure or the ability to experience it), flat affect, and avolition (loss of motivation). She had a history of depression and bizarre behaviour (details unavailable) that were exacerbated by the loss of her daughter prior to her diagnoses. Her presenting symptoms were primarily pain in her "phantom leg" (from the below the left knee amputation), all over body itching, paranoiac delusions around washing/bathing and changing her clothes, a need to be isolated, and lack of desire to engage with others (Information extracted from case notes, referenced to DSM-IV-TR, 2000).

Two years after the amputation, Y continued to experience phantom limb pain and later, a quite prominent symptom of itchy skin. When she was experiencing this itch, it was quite prominent in her phantom limb. It was also clearly present during periods when she spoke of her child and would cry out, "my leg, my leg, it hurts too much. Please, please it hurts ..."

Y would speak to people, but was suspicious and would only give answers that she felt were necessary. She would repeatedly shrug her left shoulder, which seemed to be an involuntary movement when she was approached and could be assumed to be an action (a form of a "tick" triggered by stress) that waylaid her anxiety of having to interact with others. Y would sit in her wheelchair singing to herself appearing oblivious to her environment, until someone asked her how she was. She would laugh if the person speaking to her laughed. As if she was imitating the person—however her laugh was without affect. She would look at them suspiciously then cry out, "my leg, my leg, it hurts too much. Please, please it hurts ..." She would continue to speak in the same tone saying, "My daughter, my daughter gone, please it hurts." It was as if she felt that she was expected to have a complaint about her health. The "ailment" seemed to be most easily expressed in terms of pain and the most obvious cause was her missing leg. There was, no doubt, that she was experiencing some sort of sensations in her phantom and explained it as pain although there may also have been the discomfort of pain, as is inevitable in phantom leg syndrome. The expression of *having pain* seemed to be her expression of *suffering* or of *being in pain.* Although, there were period of time, throughout the day, when she would complain of pain in "the leg that is not there", she refused medication due to a paranoia that she would be poisoned.

The neurotic symptoms that Y displayed were those of shrugging her shoulder, crying out repeatedly about her leg and her daughter, but of most significant interest was her scratching her skin to relieve an allusive "itch".

The symptom of itching and scratching was so prominent that it presented as some form of gratification or satisfaction of desire. In Freud's (1905) *Three Essays on the Theory of Sexuality* there is an interesting explanation of the presence and role of an "itch". In order to again achieve a previous satisfaction, a desire or compulsion to repeat a certain behaviour is present—due to past experience:

> [T]he state of being in need of a repetition of the satisfaction reveals itself in two ways: by a peculiar feeling of tension, possessing, rather, the character of unpleasure, and by a sensation of itching or stimulation which is centrally conditioned and projected on to the peripheral erotogenic zone. We can therefore formulate a sexual aim in another way: it consists in replacing the projected sensation of stimulation in the erotogenic zone by an external stimulus which removes that sensation by producing a feeling of satisfaction. (p. 184)

I realise here that it is no surprise that an itch is a result of a build-up of energy resulting in a need for relief. In recent research, it has been discovered that the sensation of itch and that of pain run on common neural pathways. There is progress toward further investigation of itching as it has been found to follow in the footsteps of chronic pain. Studies so far have shown that severe and chronic itch "disrupts sleep and other aspects of life and carries a heavy economic and social burden" (Carsten, 2009, p. 73). We need to note that as with pain, itch plays positive as well as negative roles. It could act as a warning as well as cause extensive exacerbation of other problems such an increase in pain and disruption in day-to-day life (ibid.). However, the feeling of satisfaction gained from relieving an itch by scratching is undeniable.

It is undeniable that *Jouissance* (Lacan, 1992) with its sexual etymology connotes the pleasure inherent in pain and the pain of too much pleasure. Tickling and sexual climax are two examples that testify to the impossibility of satisfaction. The aim of the *pleasure principle* (Freud, 1920g) is to work toward maintaining equilibrium (to keep pleasure to a minimum) and therefore, a "prohibition" of *Jouissance*. Beyond the limits of the pleasure principle and beyond the limits of pleasure that the subject can bare is pain. Beyond this limit, pleasure becomes pain or an experience of "pleasurable pain". *Jouissance*, then, is this "suffering" and "expresses the paradoxical satisfaction that the subject derives from his symptom, or to put it another way, the suffering that he derives from his own satisfaction" (Evans, 2005, pp. 91–92) (Freud's "primary gain from illness").

There is evidence in the case of Y, who would scratch herself until her skin was raw, but would not stop until, suddenly she would begin to giggle and then be distracted by the activities around her. She would say that she has an itch and that her body is "itchy" and that she needs to "scratch". It seems as if this behaviour was part of her psychosis as well as the build-up and release of scratching the itch, seemed to serve as a means to sexual gratification. During these periods she was oblivious to where she was or who was present, completely absorbed in this activity that she repeated several times during the day. It needs to be noted that at the end of this activity Y's body was notably marked and sore from the exertion. Whatever discomfort or pain she experienced from the vigorous scratching seemed to be a means to a pleasurable end!

Freud stated that in neurosis, the piece of reality that is cut off "takes flight" and in psychosis that piece of reality is "remodelled". Neurosis does not disavow the reality, it only ignores it; however, psychosis disavows it and tries to replace it. Here, then it is "no longer *autoplastic* but *alloplastic*" (1924b, pp. 184–185).

Autoplastic (*repair the internal environment with matter from another part of that environment*) and alloplastic (*to replace or change the internal environment*) are terms used in psychoanalysis to explain the interaction with the external reality in an attempt to repair or replace a part of the internal reality. These terms can also be referred to the term *plasticity* used to describe a process that occurs (not exclusively) within phantom limb syndrome (pain), the brain's ability to reorganise itself in order to maintain the body/self integrity (Ramachandran, 1994) as discussed earlier in this chapter.

Analysis

It seemed that Y's experience of phantom limb pain and that of the loss of her child had somehow become entangled in her psychic make-up and were as one. I propose here that the phantom limb pain was an attempt at repairing the pain of the reality of her loss. The phantom limb can also be applied as a metaphor for her internal experiences of *being in pain*. I would go so far as to venture that not only her phantom limb but also her itch were types of screen memories created by her mind as an attempt to repair the breach in her psychological processing. Her sense of loss was thus expressed, as was her desire for sexual gratification and an autoerotic act of (infantile, narcissistic) self-preservation.

The fear of being poisoned was a fear of punishment from the external world, an obsessive thought process, for the loss of her daughter. Y had clearly created another reality to satisfy the loss of the real world which was evidenced in her rationalisations. Her paranoia, it seemed, replaced her feeling of guilt and loss.

As long as she was not compelled to engage, she was content, clearly, with herself. She was engaged in her *private world*. There were times when she sang and laughed, to herself. At other times, she would experience *itching* that she had throughout the day, at various intensities. During periods of heightened anxiety she would scratch herself until her skin was quite sore, clearly distressed, and no amount of creams or other solutions (she mostly refused all treatments) would placate her need to scratch herself. There had been several medical investigations to rule out any physical or physiological problems or illness. Upon observation, it was clear that she found a sort of comfort, even pleasure, in scratching. As in the case of someone being bitten by a mosquito and the resulting need to scratch the area, her expression would turn from distress to relief.

The itch, I propose, is a form of, and part of, the physical as well as the emotional phantom pain that Y experienced. The only relief she seemed to attain was by scratching. Y had been known to express that she liked to scratch herself whether or not she feels an itch. At times, it had been observed that Y laughed and giggled as she scratched her body. At these times, she would refuse to engage and would ignore any interaction or conversation. In these instances, the scratching appeared to be a route to sexual gratification. I would argue that Y had found a spot on her upper body to relieve the itching in her phantom leg. It could also be that Y scratched herself to provoke pain in order to elicit a pleasurable sensation. It appeared that relieving the "itch" brought Y a degree of pleasure in the form of release of built-up energy, such as an orgasm, or as scratching an itchy spot does where also there is a build-up of energy and release (if you get the right spot!). This, I suggest, is a good example of pain, in the form of an itch, being used in the service of self-gratification and pleasure—a desire for self-preservation within an ego-cathexis. Y created her own object in creating pain (an itch) that she used to gain pleasure.

Y was also diagnosed with was depression; however, it seemed that this was due to the fact that she did not wish to engage with anyone, except when she was crying about the pain in her leg and the loss of her daughter, not wanting to bathe and change her clothes, and her paranoia around being poisoned by the medication, as well as the fear of bathing as if it was a fear of losing control to others who may take something away from her. She also refused to eat which may have been part of her paranoia. However, this did not appear to be a primary concern considering the fact that she ate very well when her friend brought food for her and that her weight was stable. Her crying out was only under the circumstances discussed above. I propose that this apparent state of depression was her wish to be left alone, and a symptom of her psychosis. She would only speak to someone if she was in need of something—such as assistance with her wheelchair and being wheeled to another area. She was happy to engage with herself and to be "cut" off from reality.

Y had created a reality within certain memory traces that were seemingly distorted; however, it seemed to be a way for her to rationalise her fears. For example, she lived in a world where she was a "slave". She said that her family before her were slaves and did not bathe themselves so she would not either. She stated that she had read about this when she was in school and in other books. On those occasions when her carers succeeded in convincing her that this was necessary for good hygiene, as well as to avoid further infections, she would be quite upset and would insist on putting on her soiled clothing.

She refused to discuss the issue further as the distress of having to "give up" her clothing was unbearable and she could not comprehend why people wished to "make her change". Y wished to maintain some level of control over her life and the "world" she found herself in.

When attempts were made to bring the reality of the situation to Y, she retaliated with aggression, as this presented a threat to *her reality*.

Her reaction was an effort to ward of further trauma from her external environment and what remained was the reality of the phantom of her past trauma—her need to itch and *be in pain*. This was her experience in reality as she knew it. Her narcissistic existence was an effort toward self-preservation.

Due to her disconnection with reality, and the lack of desire for relating to her external world, I assumed that Y was content to find pleasure without any inhibitions pertaining to the external world. Her scratching herself was a perverse manifestation of her creating an "object" through which to gain pleasure. It evidences the subject's relationship with pain as it exists within her perception of the reality of pain within her perverse relationship to reality. I propose that pain, in Y's case, the "itch", is an object libidinally cathected by her (the subject).

Y was a person who had a good sense of humour when she was lucid and knew how to joke, particularly about her situation. She would say, for example, "I wanta scratch de leg dat's not dere but you see dere is no leg, why me think dere is a leg", and she would then laugh at her own joke. At first it seemed to be a sort of pathetic statement, yet we can relate it to Freud's statement:

> Like jokes and the comic, humor has something liberating about it; but it also has something of grandeur and elevation [...]. The grandeur in it clearly lies in the triumph of narcissism, the victorious assertion of the ego's invulnerability. The ego refuses to be distressed by the provocation of reality, to let itself be compelled to suffer. It insists that it cannot be affected by the traumas of the external world. It shows, in fact, that such traumas are no more than occasions for it to gain pleasure. (1927d, p. 162)

According to this, Y certainly appeared to laugh at her predicament seemingly not affected by its tragedy and behaved in such a manner as to avoid the trauma of her situation. It was also observed that Y would begin to scratch when under stressful situations. Within Y's psychotic state it was clear that the ego was detached from reality and saw only its own need to be isolated from the external world. It perceived the external world's demand as intrusive resulting in her becoming paranoid that manifested in aggressive behaviour. The scratching seemed to make her focus on her body as the object of her pleasure, an ego-cathexis, and gave her a certain degree of control over the stressful or painful moments. She scratched, creating the "itch" as a perverse object to be used to gain some kind of pleasurable relief. This appeared to be an autoerotic behaviour that could be traced back to the stage of infantile sexuality and behaviour such as thumb sucking to relieve the loss of the object and an attempt at self-preservation (Freud, 1905, p. 170).

When Y was initially engaged in conversation, she would begin with saying, "pain, pain, all de time pain. It never stops. In me leg—de one dat is not dere." She would look at the other person as if she was waiting for a reaction. At the same time, she would refuse her pain medication or any other suggestions to relieve the "pain". Y's pain was her only relief from the reality of the loss of her daughter, her home, her limb, and her independence in her community. This, it appeared, was her suffering. However, due to her psychosis, the reality of her sense of being in pain and suffering had been distorted, creating paranoia and a need to protect herself at all cost.

Conclusion

In conclusion, I would like to recapitulate my proposal that the psychomatrix is specific to emotions and feelings generated by memories of experiences imprinted in the matrices. The psychomatrix and neuromatrix work together to create a working unity of the body, brain, and mind.

A breach in the psychological, as well as neurological, protective mechanisms creates a state of being in pain or suffering—that is, the matrices work in the service of trying to maintain the unity of the whole. The signatures modulate or reconstitute stimuli that enter the matrices to respond to experiences and promote learning. In Y's case, the reorganising of her *psychomatrix* was to respond to her internal and external world as far as her psychotic state of mind allowed.

Dimensions of perversion and fetishism are present in these circumstances as the ego attempts to re-establish the emotional whole self. The ego cathected with the self uses pain to overcome the sense of loss of the whole (self and reality). Pain, in the form of an itch, appears to be used as a defence mechanism to cover up the breach in the loss of reality within psychosis. It is the substitute that fills the space created by the loss in an effort toward self-preservation and sexual satisfaction.

The phantom limb (pain) syndrome has a neurological as well as psychological significance and is also acknowledged as a phenomenon that could explain certain brain, as well as, mind functions.

I have argued that this phenomenon is a metaphor for the experience of *being in pain* or *suffering*. I have applied it to fetishism within perversion—such as disavowal. The space left by an emotional loss is filled by pain. Pain, within anxiety, is also a reminder of that which is lost. Therefore, pain is an object constructed from the subject's desire to fill the space caused by a loss. Suffering is a consequence of loss and the patient may feel pain, purposefully, inflicted by an external source. Pain felt as a "thing" inflicted rather than suffered can also be inflicted by a person on himself (Abel-Hirsch, 2006, p. 101).

As a thing that is apart from one's physical or psychological being, it is assumed to be easier to get rid of or to cut out. As an object, it can also be manipulated and used to fulfil certain desires of pleasure and self-preservation. The subject-pain relationship is the desire for pleasure and self-preservation and exists within the emotional sphere. I propose that the subject-pain relationship is an inseparable state, creating the premise for all human behaviour. As an object, distance is created where pain becomes the desired and *being in pain* thus, may be used as a defence against a traumatic situation.

Pain, I have proposed, is the acknowledgement as well as denial of that which is desired, a misrepresentation central to an understanding of perversion and arises from quite a specific mechanism in which contradictory versions of reality are allowed to coexist simultaneously (Abel-Hirsch, 2006, p. 102).

To conclude this chapter it is important to stress that the neuromatrix and the psychomatrix work in tandem to create a sense of existence—physical and psychological. The significance of the subject-pain relationship is key in gaining an understanding of his existence and identity, in relation to his own reality, as well as in relation to others.

Phantom pain has been seen to be a type of chronic pain syndrome and over time changes in intensity and shape. However, as with any chronic pain, its complexity lies in the many dimensions of the psychological and emotional system of the mind.

CHAPTER FIVE

Chronic pain syndrome

Introduction

Chronic pain implies that a pain has been noxious and persistently present for some time. How did chronic pain become such an attention seeking entity in the midst of society? And not only in the Western world but clearly and sadly throughout the world, particularly in developing countries where pain medicine and pain management are not a priority for the bureaucratic systems that govern health services (Sessle, 2007, p. 27; Rajagopal, 2009, pp. 312–318).

Chronic pain, like the phantom limb, is a neurologically and psychologically controversial subject area. It is a topic that has been researched from many different perspectives and the conclusions arrived at continue to leave the debate ongoing over the questions of "where exactly is the pain situated in the body?" and "why can it not be treated successfully, so that the patient can maintain a pain free existence?" It is like a "phantom" being tracked. In the last fifty or so years researchers have attempted to focus in on certain characteristics and personalities of certain demographic groups of individuals, who suffer with similar types of chronic pain, in a variety of circumstances. At the same time there is a movement towards a wider perspective of causation and etymology of pain which remains, even after the *acute pain* has been treated.

> Studies based on psychological theories attempted to show that patients with intractable pain shared certain personality characteristics which predisposed them to pain. Underlying this body of work were the following assumptions: (a) pain is caused by either organic or psychological factors; (b) pain which does not correspond to known physical pathology is psychological in origin: and (c) patients with undiagnosed intractable pain are a psychologically homogeneous group. In the past 10–15 years, the dualistic conceptions and linear causal views which buttressed these assumptions have been cogently challenged. During the same time, research has been criticized for weak methodology, inconsistent findings, biased interpretations of data, and questionable conceptualizations. (Gamsa, 1994, p. 17)

However, in spite of the controversy, and for the purposes of my book, it is significant to keep in mind the "assumptions" as stated in the quote above. Not because there has been concrete evidence that chronic pain is psychological but because the sufferer of chronic pain, as equally with physical pain, suffers psychologically and emotionally. There are those who present with symptoms of chronic pain with a desire to find an organic cause—or evidence—in an effort to obtain medical relief and/or, as evidenced in research, for other motives. However, I also know of people, in the general public, who present to their doctors with conditions other than physical pain. Investigations usually lead to and uncover levels of stress and anxieties that disrupt daily activities—not necessarily as a chronic pain in the *physical domain*. If untreated, though, this type of pain, no matter what the reason or motive, manifests itself within the many dimensions of the individual's life. Pain research has progressed to find some, quite, convincing indications, primarily, that psychological factors commonly manifest as chronic pain syndrome, such as fibromyalgia, and is not less actual or painful than pain from physical, internal, or external sources. Though, the debate continues to be viewed through controversial lenses as it evades definitive explanations. Chronic pain, such as fibromyalgia, raises speculations into the motivating factors of the subject's complaints, and presents many environmental—psychological, physical, cultural, and developmental—complications for aetiology and diagnoses.

The above assumptions seem controversial particularly that of those who suffer chronic pain are "a psychologically homogenous group". There are studies that do verify this assertion, on the one hand, and other studies that show that this may not be the case. Either way it is clear that chronic pain, even though it may have an organic or physical origin, becomes established in the psychological and emotional systems of the mind, at varying degrees, due to each individual's innate psychological matrix, and as Flor (2009) states, that "learning influences subjective, behavioural, neuro-psychological, and biochemical aspects of pain that outlast the phase of acute pain and may contribute to an enhanced experience of chronic pain" (p. 234).

It has been shown that those who are living with physical pain such as that caused by arthritis, rheumatism, cancers, and other diseases experience pain at varying subjective intensities contingent upon his emotional and psychological state. Clauw and Abdin (2009) state:

> [The] role of psychological distress in triggering FM and related illnesses has been accepted almost as dogma for some time, based on the observations of high level of distress among these patients, the abnormalities observed in the stress response systems among these patients, and the general feeling of "stress" experienced by physicians caring for these patients. (p. 256)

There have been innumerable studies conducted to find specific links between psychological stress to a variety of related conditions such as those caused by motor accidents, HIV, osteoarthritis, and catastrophic events such as terrorism and other man-made and other disasters, to name only a few. The controversies, however, are an indication of the sensitivities of this topic particularly as it appears to be a problem that is on the increase in societies around the world.

Learning and plasticity seem to have a great influence in the progression of chronic pain. It has been show in research that the development of chronic pain syndrome is a learned process (Flor, 2009; Huber et al., 2010). The meaning behind the pain and what is causing it is also seen to be significant. Therefore, the assumptions, of course, are drawn from evidence gained from previous investigations and in an effort to narrow the field of research.

These scientific attempts will, of course, continue in order to find a concrete, *scientific* structure within which to diagnose and treat pain as a disease.

The first two assumptions appear to be stating the obvious. All three assumptions seem to be the "unmentionable" and unvoiced due to the politics of "judgmentalism" (Rogers, 2004). However, there are researchers who have taken a brave stance and gone beyond the irritation of chronic pain complaints to look at what is behind the complaints. In the spirit of "active listening" (Rogers, 2004), chronic pain is now being seen as a symptom of something that runs deeper and through every dimension of an individual's life. As Rey (1995) states:

> [W]hen pain is intense and persistent or simply chronic, it always involves the entire being. It does not only limit itself to the painful region, but it is the whole person as an individual entity who then becomes affected as a result; his entire personality becomes doleful and his intellect becomes dulled. (p. 3)

We understand the assumptions are referring to a group of individuals who are essentially alike and who have similar psychological traits and characteristics, and who present in a similar manner. Albeit there are certain groups of people who can be categorised for the sake of scientific research, we suggest that chronic pain or pain that is rooted in the psychological and emotional system, is evasive due to its subjective complexity. The meaning behind one's pain is what is in question and meaning is not something that can be categorised. It may be like saying that those who have issues with their mothers or those who step on ants have unconscious, perverse, sadistic tendencies! This pretty much includes everyone.

Within the context of this book, it is important to keep in mind that I am proposing that any one individual has the potential to develop what is known as chronic pain syndrome. Pain that persists beyond an organic cause or noxious external stimuli is pain that each one of us has. The assumptions, of course, we need to understand are an effort to narrow the field of research in an attempt to find a structure within which to diagnose and treat pain as a disease. For example, the July/August 2010 issue of the *Journal of Pain Research & Management* published a research project conducted by Huber, Kunz, Artelt, and Lautenbacher. The research was "to assess maladaptive attentional and emotional mechanisms of pain processing and their related factors". It was a highly scientific research using "a structural equation approach". A group of ninety-two healthy young men and women was used to measure maladaptive, attentional, and emotional pain processing. This was done using a set of self-report measures. "The comprehensive set of predictor variables included measures of affective and bodily distress" such as depression, anxiety and somatisation. Not surprisingly, the conclusions indicated that anxiety and depression, as well as somatisation, contributed to this maladaptive behaviour:

> Pain hypervigilance, pain-related anxiety and pain catastrophizing have been found to be strongly intercorrelated constructs, and are all part of contemporary avoidance models of pain. [...] refer to attentional and emotional processes, through which certain individuals focus exclusively on as well as exaggerate the threat value of pain or pain-related stimuli. [...] might predispose these individuals to develop or maintain chronic pain. (p. 229)

Research is still lacking in evidence identifying potentially related factors that might cause this behaviour. Why some individual do and others do not show maladaptive processing of pain is a question that lies unanswered. Nevertheless, what is relevant to this book is that all individuals display certain behaviours according to their own subjective perception of their pain. And further, I argue, this behaviour is contingent upon the relationship that exists between the subject and his pain. The behaviour is also indicative of the impact that this relationship has on their sense of identity and their sense of existence.

Chronic pain such as fibromyalgia, I argue, is evasive as it is based in the emotive sphere of the individual's functioning, be it physical or psychological. As discussed in previous chapters, pain from any source of experience becomes imprinted within the unconscious. Here, becoming part of the conglomerate of pain, it impacts behaviour through the mechanisms of the psychomatrix within which is created patterns or psychosignatures specific to emotional pain. I will present a scenario that will be discussed further in this chapter, as with the previous chapter, and will act as an example to evidence my theory.

So far, the mystery of pain and the questions of who really suffers and why remains, as science continuous on its quest for a concrete diagnosis. It is, seemingly, the demand of society in general—"Here is my problem, it is a pain, fix it."—to discuss the possibility of pain being the symptom of a deeper, underlying psychological or emotional issue means that the "quick fix" of pain medication, or acquisition of another demand, is delayed. It could also mean, for example, that the attention gained from "being ill" is taken away, or the justification for taking extended time off from work is removed, or a carer may feel that they are no longer "needed". I will argue that as with the issue of perversion, we all have the capacity to fall into these circumstances however, what influences the aetiology of chronic pain is motive and memory coupled with the subject-pain relationship. It is not the sensation or feeling pain or *having pain* but the *being in pain*. It is the experience within the emotive relational sphere of desire.

A discussion in the journal *Pain* (1981), on the subject of tertiary gain and chronic pain, examined the opinion of doctors and other medical professionals who were working with chronic pain patients. They were recognising the existence of factors, other than observable physical factors, which influenced these patients and maintained their complaints of pain. It goes on to suggest that research in the psychiatric field has identified occurrences of "primary or secondary gain" identified by Dansak (1973).

Primary gain occurs in the psychological mechanism as a defence mechanism against "unacceptable affect or conflict". Secondary gain is the relational or "environmental advantage supplied by a symptom(s)". "Tertiary" gain is also an interpersonal occurrence however, it is when someone else other than the patient benefits or may seek to benefit from the person's illness (Bokan et al., 1981, p. 331).

The discussion paper concludes:

> It is imperative that those dealing with pain patients include in the evaluation the social context of the patient. The social context includes not only the patient's family, work, etc., but also the physician or health care system. Gain is a useful way to conceive and communicate certain aspects that are active in the situation, exacerbation, complication, evaluation, and rehabilitation of chronic pain. (ibid., p. 335)

This indeed makes sense, as in diagnosing any illness or problem and would be beneficial to evaluate a person from a systemic perspective; however, *pain* does not go away. It seems that chronic pain, as we see in fibromyalgia and the phantom limb syndrome, remain true as part of the mechanism of defence.

Historically psychological perspectives have been applied erratically to chronic pain without an obvious physical or organic basis. However, during the second half of the last century, research into the problem of chronic pain made a decisive turn due to many reasons, however, mainly due to various, but persistent, opinions, of several researchers, about the impact of emotional and psychological factors on this topic.

Gamsa's (1994) research into this area has examined Merskey and Spear's (1967) comprehensive historical compilation of the literature on the psychological aspects of pain from as far back as the 1700s. Scientists such as Livingston (1943), Szasz (1957), Engel (1959), Wall (1979), and Melzack and Wall (1986, 1996) have contributed to research into the emotional, psychological, and psychoanalytical implications of chronic pain.

There are other investigators such as Pontalis (1981), Clyman (1991), Morris (1993), Rey (1995), Akhtar (2000), Flor (2009), Clauw and Ablin (2009), and Huber et al. (2010) who continue to examine various other perspectives on chronic pain or pain that persists beyond an acute phase, and have examined the dimensions of psychological suffering. The question that continues to arise is: What is the purpose of chronic pain?

I start with the premise that "[P]ain is an effraction, it supposes the existence of limits: limits of the body, limits of the ego, it brings about an internal discharge, which could be called an implosion effect" (Pontalis, 1981, p. 196). And, as recently stated by Gamsa (1993), "[i]t is now generally recognized that psychological factors play an important role in chronic pain" (p. 5).

When considering the psychoanalytic perspective of pleasure inherent in pain or pleasure hidden in suffering we can trace the psychological and emotional aspects of chronic pain in a subject in analysis where "we find suffering and the movement of the treatment consists in discovering and showing by what detours this suffering is produced, induced, unconsciously sought by the individual himself, in order to obtain a premium of pleasure in some other intrapsychic place" (Pontalis, 1981, p. 197).

Here again, I propose that an emotive relational aspect may be detected within the dimensions of desire where pain is the desired object through which a "premium of pleasure" may be achieved.

Elements of chronic pain

Chronic pain is pain that does not go away. The protective value of an acute pain that alerts us of tissue damage or the risk of damage or a warning to avoid certain situations where this damage can occur, is lost in chronic pain. It is defined as symptoms of unremitting pain that last for six months or more. There are a variety of aspects of chronic pain which are not yet understood. Chronic pain may be associated with a variety of circumstances, illnesses, and disabilities such as phantom limb syndrome, cancer and arthritis. There are some types of chronic pain that begin after an injury and persist over time. Other types of chronic pain include fibromyalgia and neuropathic pain. In some cases, the cause of chronic pain is known, however more commonly the cause is not known. There is an increasing number of chronic pain suffers, according to statistics from research funded and conducted by organi-sations such as the International Association for the Study of Pain. The direct and indirect costs associated with chronic pain are staggering. Chronic pain affects both sexes; however, it has been found that the rates are slightly higher in women. Chronic pain also has the aspect of psychological problems such as anxieties and depression and can disrupt sleep, reduce energy, and impair work and social activities, and have a negative impact on financial security, and in some cases it can contribute to alcohol or drug abuse. Chronic pain has also been seen to be a culprit in disrupting marital and family relationships (Sessle, 2007; Glombiewski, 2010; Flor, 2009).

Pain is invisible and draws the individual into a clouded space. The chronic sufferer can feel alone and isolated and misunderstood and many find that the legitimacy of their pain is questioned. Then there are those who believe that the pain is all in their heads which, indeed, has a ring of truth because the brain (as well as the mind) is very actively involved in this experience—physical or phenomenological or psycho-logical. We know, through research, that what happens in one's mind is inherently tied to what happens in one's brain and body, as well as the other way round. Given the impact pain can have on quality of life it is not surprising that more than a quarter of people who experience chronic pain also experience significant depression or anxiety. Other areas where deficits have been found are attention, memory, mental flexibility such as problem solving and information processing speed—independent of mood. The primary problem, with chronic pain, such as fibromyalgia, is that often sensory input is absent as with the pain in a phantom limb. Chronic pain has a developmental and historical aspect that has been recently explored and evidence shows that it is "determined to a large extent by learning and memory processes" (Flor, 2009, p. 221).

Of course, the above conclusion is an extension of Freud's (1895) research in his *Project* (1950a) as well as Melzack's (1993) neuromatrix theory. Our innate abilities are modulated by our experiences and thus determine the processes of learning and memory. Since pain is the primary and vital element in our development and functioning, it is feasible that it is processed, not only through our neurological and psychological systems but, also throughout our emotional system. Human behaviour, as Freud first "scientifically" acknowledged over a hundred years ago, revolves around human relations. The pain that is the cause and effect of these human relations is the primary focus as it is the core of all interactions. The subject-pain relationship is derived from human relationships from the emotional premise of desire.

The experience of chronic pain is a desire for the lost object. Pain fills that void and remains as a constant reminder, but it also becomes the object within and a means to gain pleasure.

Chronic pain, a chronic suffering

My argument is that chronic pain is the phantom of past trauma, just as I have discussed is the case in the phantom limb syndrome. The difference is that instead of pain being in a part of the body that does not exist pain is experienced in areas of the body that very much exist. The uncanny notion is that pain of this sort, in most cases, is not actually caused by anything physical that has sent a message to the brain to interpret or register as physical pain. However, in spite of this the individual experiences *having pain* in a part of the body and determined to find a remedy.

Chronic pain has sometimes been diagnosed as a hysterical symptom of a conversion disorder. That is to say that a past, unresolved sexual trauma is converted to or manifests as a physical pain. Individuals who suffer chronic pain have also been labelled as 'neurotic' when there is no apparent organic cause. Freud (1905e) wisely proposed an organic subtlety in the psychological and chronic pains of hysteria: "[N]o one, probably, will be inclined to deny the sexual function the character of an organic factor, and it is the sexual function that I look upon as the foundation of hysteria and of the psychoneuroses in general" (p. 113).

In my practice, I have come across several patients experiencing chronic headaches and lower back pain with no apparent physical cause. For example, a forty-five-year-old woman who had a very sheltered upbringing and who looked after her aging parents until they died had complained of chronic headaches or migraines for a number of years. She had admittedly never been in an intimate relationship and devoted her time to works of charity. Her conversations revealed that as a child she had wanted to get married and have children; however, due to her parents' illness and caring for them, this wish had not materialised. Sex outside of a marriage had always been an unthinkable thing, which she had abstained from. Her conversations revolved around her headaches, the process that she went through, every time, to detect them and manage them and what she did to manage them, which was injecting herself with a strong migraine medication. She carried the injections in her bag so that she could have them at hand if needed.

This patient admitted that she never drank water unless she was at home and near a toilet, as she was fearful of needing to pass urine and not having access to a clean toilet.

It was discovered, however, that she was suffering dehydration which in turn affected the functioning of her (brain) electrolytes, causing her to have pain in her head. In spite of this finding, my patient insisted that it was more than that because she believed that she drank enough water and never felt thirsty. She further insisted that she needed her injection.

She had stated at one point, "as soon as I feel a headache coming on I must get the needle ready. As soon as the pain gets to a certain point I give myself the injection and straight away I feel relief." It was curious this explanation as it had a prominent bearing on her desire to find a release from her "headache" which I believe was rooted in her childhood desire to marry and her thwarted sexual desire. Sexuality and sex, being such a taboo topic in her life, was converted to a migraine, maintained by her lack of hydration and momentarily satisfied by the injection.

The subject-pain relationship is clear—pain is the object that my patient sought in order to gain a measure of pleasure and self-preservation. It is therefore correct that the "psychological basis of pain is often subtle and complex, with multiple interacting mechanisms that preclude simple causal labels (Pilowsky, 1994)" (Melzack & Wall, 2008, p. 256).

Pain has its own language and each individual who has experienced the presence of his pain, expresses it in his own way. "Whether it is a cry, a sob, or a tensing of features [...] coloured by subjective considerations" (Rey, 1995, pp. 4–5),

> [t]he relationship between physical pain and emotional distress has been recognised for some time. In Genesis Chapter Three, when the pain of child-birth is inflicted upon the human race, the Bible state: "In sorrow thou shalt bring forth children", indicating an interchangeable relationship between pain and sorrow. Although pain and emotional distress are inextricably linked by scientists, clinicians, and lay persons, this relationship is much more complicated than simple cause and effect. (Clauw & Ablin, 2009, p. 245)

Suffering or *being in pain* as we have previously discussed is rooted in the emotional and psychological system of our unconscious mind. From the memories of representations of experiences here, suffering tends to influence one's life and its processes, such as, learning to survive and procreate, instinctually. However, apart from this psychological aspect suffering or being in pain has a phenomenological proponent—the conscious mind. The duality of the existence of pain is necessary in discussing chronic pain syndrome as it was when discussing the phantom limb syndrome. The link between pain and the emotions and psychological system has been established, as evidenced from research. However, what evades knowledge and comprehension is why it exists, where is it situated, and how it can be eliminated, managed or treated.

Research continues to facilitate further knowledge and understanding of this phenomenon and has discovered that there are a variety of treatments indicated for chronic pain such as fibromyalgia. However, again, there is not one that affords a lasting relief. As with the phantom limb, the pain returns.

Recent research by Glombiewski et al. (2010) on chronic pain treatments evidences this and the necessity for ongoing research. It discusses that psychological interventions are known to be effective in treating various pain disorder such as chronic pain in fibromyalgia. However, only a few systematic reviews on this subject exist. In sum, it remains unclear whether psychological treatments, such as cognitive behavioural therapy, are effective in reducing symptoms of chronic pain such as fibromyalgia (pp. 280–281).

Pharmacological treatments have been used with some success; however, these, as well, fail to be long-term remedies. It is increasingly recognised that pharmacological along with psychological interventions are needed, in a balanced programme, in order to treat chronic pain to some degree of success. Nevertheless, in spite of there being a variety of interventions being used the symptoms of chronic pain—including unremitting pain in various parts of the body—anxieties, depression, fatigue, demotivation for activity, and so on return.

Recent research has evidenced that chronic pain is largely determined by learning processes that are accompanied by "plastic changes at multiple levels of the nervous system".

> A fundamental distinction can be made between implicit (or nondeclarative) and explicit (or declarative) memory processes. Implicit memory processes refer to changes in behaviour that develop—often unconsciously—as a consequence of experience. [...] nonassociative learning processes such as, habituation and sensitization, as well as associative processes such as, operant and respondent conditioning. Explicit learning [...] semantic and episodic memory processes that rely on the conscious reproduction of an encoded memory item. (Flor, 2009, p. 222)

Implicit memory is the more significant, it seems, of the two, as pain has a high biological relevance, with roots in human evolution and survival—needing automatic, instinctual decision making ability such as in the "fight or flee" scenarios.

In 1895, Freud's *Project* indicated a similar hypothesis as well as that emotion and memory operate within a seamless system. Summarising a report by Rapaport (1950a), it seems that an experience is imprinted in the memory, but not before it is influenced by previously stored material. There are instinctual impulses which originate in the systems of the unconscious that are triggered and impact thought and behaviour. Thus, "selective forces of instinctual origin and process of habituation are interlaced in memory function, producing [...] impenetrable memory" (Pribram & Gill, 1976, p. 70).

Pribram and Gill (1976) further explained Freud's theory from the *Project* stating that memory and motive are both processes based on selective facilitation of impermeable neurons. As with implicit and explicit memory processes he hypothesised that memories are the "retrospective aspects of facilitation; and motives the prospective aspect" (p. 70).

Therefore, learning and conditioning take place as a result of innate abilities and experience, however according to Freud's theory, "experiences can be distorted by the subsequent development of the drive system at puberty". Motive and memory are, then, linked to provide the structure of the "wish" which is a fundamental psychoanalytical contribution (ibid., pp. 70–71).

Chronic pain, I propose stems from these mechanisms of memory and motive which are influenced by the emotional workings of the mind. Learning is based on memory and motive and manifests in certain behaviours. As Flor (2009) suggests, "implicit learning processes change an individual's behaviour without his or her conscious awareness" and present challenges in the development of effective interventions (p. 222).

We know from research that the emotional state of an individual has an impact and may generate or exacerbate the state of pain chronicity. Psychoanalytical perspectives propose that pain that exists without an organic explanation is a "defence against unconscious psychic conflict where it is displaced onto the body" (Gamsa, 1994, p. 6). Psychological pain is more difficult to explain and evidence than pain situated in a part of the body. I suggest that it is easier to say that one has a chronic pain in the lower back and other muscles that will not go away, rather than take the risk of explaining that one is traumatised from domestic violence or childhood abuse and abandonment issues. Further research suggests that those suffering with chronic pain suffer unresolved, unconscious conflicts. Pain is a manifestation of those conflicts and is:

> attributed to problems such as repressed hostility and aggression, rigid superego, guilt, resentment, defence against loss or threatened loss, early childhood deprivation or trauma, masked depression,

neuroticism, and various personality disorders (Bond & Pearson, 1969; Parkes, 1973; Lese, 1974; Hughes & Zimm, 1978; Merskey & Boyd, 1978; Swanson, 1984; Violon, 1982). (Gamsa, 1994, p. 6)

These appear to be a broad range of ideas loosely connected to psychoanalytic theory and hold the common view that emotional disturbance finds expression in pain (ibid.).

Chronic pain and the psychomatrix

My view is that the problem of chronic pain rests within the creation of the psychomatrix. We know from previous exploration that the neurological system has the propensity for plasticity, as evidenced in the phantom limb phenomenon. There is this propensity in the psychological and emotional systems as well, particularly seen in chronic pain syndrome. According to Flor (2009):

> We have shown that learning influences subjective, behavioural, neuro-physiological, and biochemical aspects of pain that outlast the phase of acute pain and may contribute to an enhanced experience of chronic pain. [...] learning history must be assessed and addressed in treatment. (p. 234)

I have proposed that our experiences, right from the beginnings of life, are imprinted on the neurological as well as the psychological mapping systems. The neuromatrix creates the neurosignature for the neurological system and parallel to this, I propose, in the unconscious, lies the psychomatrix within which is created the psychosignature. Working in tandem, they create the subject's sense of the body/mind/self unity.

As stimuli, internal or external experiences, travel through the matrices, the signatures are modulated and have an impact on responses that manifest in certain actions and behaviour. This response is in an effort to maintain the integrity of the body/self or the mind/self unities, as we have explored in the previous chapter. Due to the processes of plasticity, those areas of the matrices continue to be *aware* of either a limb or the sense of a whole emotional self and demand that the *map* maintain its integrity. Pain that remains beyond the acute phase is pain that has "moved" into that area or space of the body/self map that is attached to the image of an intact limb. In case of the mind/self map there is a similar movement to an empty space triggered by an event that threatens to bring the unconscious material into the conscious therefore, causing a sense of increased pain to fill the space. This maintains the integrity of the whole emotional self. There is now created the phantom pain which is the sense of *being in pain*. Within the empty space is pain. It is a representation of that which is lost, as well as a desire to fill that space with the same.

The case of X

The following is an example of chronic pain syndrome in a person diagnosed with fibromyalgia. Having failed to establish a particular organic cause for the unremitting pain and unsuccessful pharmacological interventions, the patient's general practitioner had referred her for psychological assessment and intervention mainly due to her symptoms of anxieties that accompanied her presentation of physical pain.

The patient X was in her early forties, married with one child. She had gained a morbid amount of weight since the birth of her child, which seemed to be a factor influencing her ongoing problem with lower back pain. She was, however, experiencing pain in various other parts of her body, such as her fingers and knee joints, and pains in her leg muscles and neck, accompanied by increased amounts of fatigue and anxiety. Over a period of about five years, she had gone through various investigations to identify the cause of her physical pain.

Historical background

Over the course of our sessions, she related the following history. She had been raised by a mother who had been supportive and encouraging. However, as X entered adulthood, this turned to criticism and expressions of disappointment, especially around the time when she began dating. She described her relationship with her mother as anxiety ridden and she felt as if nothing she did was ever going to be good enough for her. At one point she even remarked that she felt that her mother was jealous of her, due to the fact that her father was an emotionally abusive man, and that she felt that she had no option but to stay in the marriage. She stated that her "mother struggled within a loveless marriage". This hostility was at times directed toward her. She eventually moved out of her parents' home. She did not date many men but eventually fell in love with a man with whom she became pregnant. However, due to the extremely volatile situation with her mother that would have been perpetuated by the extreme differences in her partner's and her culture she decided to terminate the pregnancy and the relationship.

After a period of depression, she returned to university to complete her degree in the sciences and began her career in the public health sector. She met her present husband who was working with her at the time, and they decided to get married shortly thereafter. She disclosed that she had been married for over ten years to this man who, shortly after their child was born, started to become verbally and emotionally abusive. She was very happy to be pregnant yet she had many fears due to her advanced age at the time.

She stated that she had developed arthritis in her late teens which became worse during her pregnancy with the weight gain. She managed to lose most of the weight following the birth of her child. Yet she began to develop lower back pain. By the time I met X she had been suffering with arthritic pain as well as back pain for about ten years. A year before she came to see us she said that she had been attending a very good fitness centre and had employed a trainer, and was also seeing a nutritionist, and had finally lost all the weight. She had been looking as she did when she first got married and was "on top of the world". At presentation, though, she was not attending the fitness centre and her nutrition and exercise routines were non-existent due to the pain that had returned. She said that it had never really stopped completely but she tried "not to think of it". However, it was now to the point where she felt "evicted from her body". She worked long hours while also looking after her daughter who was nine years old. She explained how important it was for her to make sure that she looked after her daughter and her schedule was completely full with school runs morning and afternoon, daily lunches that she would have with her daughter, after school programmes, and planned weekend activities. X's friends were other children's mothers whom she met at her daughter's school during the day. Other than that, she did not seem to have any meaningful friendships.

Even though she related numerous instances where her husband was abusive towards her and her pain and distress over this, she would say that they were "working on their marriage" or "he had agreed to go to some couple's therapy". She stated that she did not understand why she had put on all this weight. She was, at the time of counselling, morbidly overweight. She complained of anxiety and fatigue and not being able to perform any of the day-to-day chores, which meant that her home, unlike in the past, "looked like a disaster zone".

Presenting symptoms

The referral from X's doctor detailed the various investigations that she had gone through and apart from a mild arthritis in her thumb joints there was no other indication of trauma or disease. Her physiology was, in general, functioning at a normal level. She had been prescribed various pain and antianxiety medication that, she reported, worked only for short periods of time. She said that the pain returned "with a vengeance".

There were five elements derived from the twenty-four sessions with X: (1) her pain was concentrated in her lower back and fingers; (2) her pain "returned with a vengeance" whenever she had had an abusive encounter with her husband; (3) her pain was peculiarly present, just as intense, when she had had an encounter with her mother; (4) she never failed to say that she had to try harder to manage her feelings towards her mother, since she could at times be supportive; and towards her husband because her marriage was very important to her. To be divorced would be a sign that she had failed and she was not going to allow this. And (5) was her insistence that she was very comfortable with her body and she pointed out that her husband, even though at times ridiculed her and was verbally abusive toward her, was happy with her just the way she was.

Analysis

X, it seems, had repressed the reality of her past traumatic life as well as being in denial about her present experiences that were equally painful. The psychological impact of this pain was manifested in symptoms of chronic pain. Gamsa's (1994) research in conjunction with Bond and Pearson (1969), Parkes (1973), Lesse (1974), Hughes and Zimin (1978), Merskey and Boyd (1978), Swanson (1984), and Violon (1982) detailed a psychoanalytic view of Freud's (1905) conversion theory. She discusses as described above, the psychoanalytic formulations, postulating the view that chronic and unremitting pain with no organic explanation is rooted in a desire to escape. It is a defence against emotional pain caused by unconscious psychic conflict. "Pain is attributed to problems such as repressed hostility and aggression, rigid superego, guilt, resentment, defence against loss or threatened loss, early childhood deprivation or trauma, masked depression, neuroticism, and various personality disorders" (pp. 3–6).

Gamsa (1994) explores Szasz's (1957) theory, proposing that the ego perceives the body as an object, such that the individual reacts to the body as something or someone outside the self. Thus, feelings are projected onto the body as though onto another person, with pain experienced as a hostile attack inflicted by the body on the suffering individual. "[P]ain also substitutes for grief over the loss of a loved one, or in the case of an amputation, for the loss of the limb."

Pain, I agree, also diverts the sufferer's attention from the real loss, and is a means to compensate for feelings of desire, guilt, and shame. Chronic pain could be considered as an expression of suffering—the individual's *being in pain*. Another theory discussed in Gamsa's (1994) article, that has been referred to previously, is Engel's (1959) who discussed the possibility of the individual developing a "'library of pain experiences' originating from (and associated with) pain provoked by peripheral stimulation" (p. 7). In this way, meaning is derived, throughout development, from the context in which it was experienced. Engle (1959) further explained that these meanings could themselves become triggers for pain without peripheral stimulation. Engel's theory speaks to Freud theory of repression as well as Melzack's original theory of the neuromatrix.

Referring back to Melzack and Wall's studies from the 1960s to the present, the problem of the experience of pain without the presence of sensory inputs does not correlate. However, Melzack's (2006) theory of the neuromatrix seems to be significant to this phenomenon as well as my proposal of the possibility of a coexisting *psychomatrix* that has been generating complex sub-signatures (modulated by the psychosignature) of emotional processes caused by a history of repressed traumas and other negative events.

X's chronic pain (fibromyalgia) was the focus of our discussions, yet it was as if pain was her only consolation. She presented arguments to oppose any suggestion of alternate treatments such as returning to her "self-care" routine of finding time to exercise, better nutrition, and spending time with her friends.

It seems, increasingly, that there is another dimension that evades identification—that of the relationship which an individual has with his pain. This relationship, considering these various hypotheses and propositions, could possibly be motivational and embedded in the emotional and memory processes of the unconscious compelling human behaviours. For example, Modell states: "The earliest psychoanalytic theories can be viewed as an explanation of the psychopathology of feelings and memory" (2003, p. 558). He also reminded us of Freud's (1895d) assumption that "hysterics suffered from reminiscences" and that the "root cause of hysteria was the memory of the trauma that acted as an unassimilated foreign body in the psyche or mental apparatus" (ibid.).

In X's case I realised that she gave an excuse (reason) for why she was not able to make changes to her life or lifestyle, which could be assumed to be a neurotic formulation. An underlying complaint was that her husband was abusively critical of her body and sexual attributes. This, we believe, was a primary factor in her weight gain, apart from the pain. She expressed her failure in her relationship by turning to food, an oral fixation, which was an attempt at self-preservation, and to fulfil her sense of loss and emptiness. She was a person with psychic suffering; she was in pain. Her pain was there as a barrier to protect herself from her repressed memories and ongoing relationship traumas. It was also a deterrent to further disappointment; and to distance herself, just enough, from the real issues to maintain control over other elements in her life that she felt needed to be sustained, such as, her career and the care of her daughter. In other words, she needed her pain in order to survive her circumstances.

It was as if X took her pain everywhere she went and needed the validation that she *had* fibromyalgia and simply "could not do certain things because it hurt too much". It was her constant companion and she derived a perverse pleasure from the attention that she gained. X was in an isolated place, alone with her pain. It was a narcissistic ego cathexis as it was clear from her narrative that she derived little or no pleasurable satisfaction from the relationship with her husband, familial and other relationships.

The relationship with her mother was one of resentment and anger as she continued to feel unsupported and unsatisfied by her. One aspect of her past which she discussed was the "lack of attention" she received from her mother who, she felt, favoured her other siblings. X felt repeatedly deprived of attention from her mother, even in her present life. She went to great lengths to explain her effort and success at finding her independence from her mother. At the same time, she expressed her anger and resentment towards her mother. She stated that she wished she could somehow "make" her mother feel how she herself felt. There was an ever-present hostility and discussion alluding to revenge.

There was another element that she did not elaborate on, however it seems to figure into her feeling of "guilt" and need for "punishment". This is the experience of the termination of her first pregnancy. Considering her strict religious upbringing this would have been forbidden and looked down upon. Her resentment towards her mother, who was not aware of this incident in X's life, was actually a hostility towards her "self". She stressed the fact that her mother was not aware of this incident, as it was none of her business. Considering the moral values she alluded to, which were part of her upbringing this seemed to be an expression of guilt and shame. Her punishment was suffering this guilt, among others in her isolation. However, it also seemed to give her some sort of sense of power, the source of which was knowledge that was hers alone. In that way no one, namely her mother could take it away from her. The pain that returned repeatedly was her escape from the repressed feelings, memories and unresolved issue from this period in her life. Could it also be that the termination represents another dimension of abuse where X puts herself in her mother's place rejecting the pregnancy as if it was herself, X? In that case, the pain that repeatedly returned was her trying to master her perception of her mother's aggressive rejection. X's relationship with her pain, then, was a desire for the lost child that represented a lost part of her *self*, her identity, and her existence. The pain not only evoked feelings of her being lost and rejected by her mother, but was also triggered repeatedly by her husband.

The only way for her to feel whole again was to have this pain in her body. As she said, "the pain is everywhere. And sometimes I feel as if my whole body aches." It was the phantom of her experiences of loss— the phantom of the lost object, her mother—and the pain of that past trauma exacerbated by her present circumstances within her marriage, and her sense of having no other options.

X's hostility, which was mainly directed at her mother, seemed to give her a sense of power as was apparent in her animated description of her own independence. She gained a perverse pleasure in discussing her physical pain as if to challenge me to change it. She admitted that she was depressed but insisted that it was only because she was in such great pain.

X *used* her pain almost as an achievement and spoke of being in pain as a reward for the traumatic experiences of her childhood. It was constructed in such a way as to be used as a fetish to ward of past trauma as well as a shield from future trauma. However, her sense of pain was also a reminder of her experiences of loss—rejection and abandonment. To take away her pain would be to dissolve her fantasy of omnipotence.

I as the analyst, in this case scenario, was in the position of *the audience* or a distant observer or witness to the omnipotence of X. The actor, X, feels in-charge of the stage and has the power to invoke the responses as she plans and wishes. I was also in the position of the mother who was now perceived to be in a passive position without the power to cause any further harm—in other words—impotent or castrated by X who was in a position to take revenge. X's pain had given her the instrument by which to demand attention from her physician but, more importantly, from her mother and her husband. She also invoked a sense of awe, as she explained how she continues to *function* in spite of this debilitating "illness".

X, it seems, brought her chronic pain complaint to sessions as an ally or an object to be manipulated to keep the real issues at bay—a resistance. It was also an effort to gain control or mastery over her past, as well as present, experiences. It was seemed clear, at times, that in resisting any suggestion at change there was an ever present sense that there was a desire to prolong the experience of the chronic pain, for the pleasure of satisfaction that it derived.

Pain as a fetish

If we pay attention to the literature on pain, including phantom pain syndrome, chronic pain syndrome, addictions, war and torture, sexual, physical and psychological abuse, there is evidence that the *associated meanings of the injuries* contribute to the intensity and chronicity of pains suffered by individuals. In the case of X, the meaning of the physical and emotional abuse that she suffered at the hands of her husband meant an invasion into her innermost sanctuary of self, her self-worth and self-image. It was an intrusion into her space as she tried desperately to keep out the noxious stimulus of his words and actions. Individuals who come in for psychotherapy are suffering a variety of such pains. Their defence mechanisms consist of varying levels of apathy and indifference, anxiety, depression, and a variety of physical pains without an organic basis—such as lower back pain, headaches, muscle fatigue, irritable bowels etc. There are many more Xs out in the world who suffer their existence.

Kierkegaard states:

> Just as a physician might say that there very likely is not one single living human being who is completely healthy, so anyone who really knows mankind might say that there is not one single living human being who does not despair a little, who does not secretly harbour an unrest, an inner strife, a disharmony, an anxiety about an unknown something or a something he does not even dare to try to know, an anxiety about some possibility in existence or an anxiety about himself, so that, just as the physician speaks of going around with an illness in the body, he walks around with a sickness, carries around a sickness of the spirit that signals its presence at rare intervals in and through an anxiety he cannot explain. (Hong & Hong, 2000, p. 357)

Pain is like a *vital sign*, as it seems to be an integral part of one's existence. X suffers the emptiness of her loss, rejection, and depleted self by constructing the only thing that will fit the space left from her loss—pain. However, it is also a reminder of the loss and instils another pain, the desire for revenge and a desire to satisfy her loss. The repeated suffering of her chronic pain confirms her desire to give new meaning to the psychological and emotional injury. Her pain is then, inevitably, such a construction. Her frantic search for a cure for her chronic pain is a symptom of her neurotic behaviour. She takes her pain with her and sits it down beside her. She points to it when she needs justification for her thoughts and actions. Her pain gives her a sense of power to think that no professional or other can know the true meaning of her pain and therefore, take it away from her. So she hangs on to it. In her neurosis, she escapes into the construction and behind her fetish.

In another scenario, if she was psychotic she would create a whole new reality that would be presented to the world as such. As Freud (1924) stated that in "neurosis a piece of reality is avoided by a sort of flight, whereas in psychosis it is remodelled". Both states are an "expression of rebellion on the part of the id against the external world' and its incapacity to "adapt itself to the exigencies of reality" (p. 185). As it is X presents with her pain looking for relief from it, though in order to get rid of her chronic pain she will need something else to fill the space. She has escaped from part of her reality behind her chronic pain therefore ignoring her reality and denying the root cause of her problems. Her protection from this part of her reality is her chronic pain. In her discussions, it is clear that her fantasy of revenge upon her mother and her husband is her sanctuary of sorts. Freud (1924) states:

> This domain has since been kept free from the demands of the exigencies of life, like a kind of "reservation", it is not inaccessible to the ego, but is only loosely attached to it. It is from this world of phantasy that the neurosis draws the material for its new wishful constructions, and it usually finds that material along the path of regression to a more satisfying real past. (p. 187)

It seems that from this place of fantasy X has constructed an object, which is her pain, namely her chronic pain, to protect her from the trauma of her childhood loss. The pain protects her from threats of re-victimisation from the trauma of her present life. It is as if her pain is her secret weapon and a vehicle for gaining power over her loss as therefore, an object which also brings her a degree of satisfaction and pleasure. In her fantasy, she can exert this power to gain the revenge that she seeks in humiliating those who humiliated her.

A long way from Freud's first postulations on perversion and fetishism, Cooper (1991) explains that Stoller (1974) has "stressed that everyone is more or less perverse". He distinguishes between "'perversion' as a diagnosis of a personality, dominated by sexual fantasy and 'perversion mechanisms' universally, applied to preserve sexual gratification against trauma". Cooper (1991) further stresses Stoller's (1974) thesis, that the core of perversion is hostility, vengeance, and fantasy. It is significant to consider Stoller's work because he combines the concept of sexuality and the earlier emphasis on castration and fetishism. In doing so, he forms a "perversion with newer concepts derived from the understanding of pre-oedipal narcissistic and safety needs and the problems of separation and individuation" (pp. 20–21). The construction of a fetish object is in aid of regaining control over the fear of passivity, to deny the experience of being helpless, and a way of taking revenge for past humiliation, rejection, abandonment and loss (ibid., p. 24).

The perspective of pain as a fetish is a key element in the formulation of my theory of the subject-pain relationship and the psychomatrix and evidences manifestations of experiences imprinted within the unconscious. Gamsa's (1994) study on pain has explored the implications of past trauma:

> In his comprehensive reviews of the literature on the effect of abuse and neglect in childhood, Roy (1982, 1985) cited several studies whose findings support a relationship between early difficulties and pain in adulthood. The findings include memories of punitive mothers and rejecting fathers (Merskey & Boyd, 1978), traumatic events in childhood and adolescence. (p. 7)

Chronic pain, from a psychoanalytic perspective, is a neurotic symptom, as can be surmised from much of this research. In repressing the unacceptable, the subject then constructs a way of protecting himself from his fears and anxieties of the real pain. However, the phantom of what is repressed is manifested in yet another pain. He, therefore, creates and maintains a "chronic pain". Chronic pain, in a way, is something that the individual has control over. He controls the occurrences, frequency, and intensity according to the anxiety provoking situation he finds himself in. It is a pain, a thing that can be used whenever he feels that it is necessary. This is similar to what Michels (2006) postulated:

> [T]he neurotic prefers to eradicate, i.e., repress, what he cannot undo, with the result that the traces of the past continue to exist as erased traces, and are actually maintained precisely because they have been erased. In paradoxical fashion, the traces have been preserved and accentuated by virtue of the fact that they have been wiped out. This process also conditions the way in which the neurotic deals with his subjective truth, which he can often approach only via a lie. (p. 83)

Therefore, I propose that the subject approaches his past trauma with his fetish which is (chronic) pain. It is that which fulfils the loss at the same time being a reminder of that which is lost. It is a defence mechanism from that which is repressed in the unconscious. Pain is that something that is inflicted on the subject himself and for his own gains.

As in the case scenario above, X brought her pain to the sessions to enact a masochistic fantasy. She was, at times, convincing enough to draw me into the game. If I showed empathy for her suffering, it was satisfaction enough. Her expressions of resentment toward her mother were presented in such a manner so as to solicit unconditional belief in the authenticity of her "illness", that subsequently brought a degree of pleasure and satisfaction to her, that her secret was safe.

Conclusion

Chronic pain becomes a disease or a disorder when the value of learning and warning produced from acute pain is lost. Research evidences that chronic pain is associated with prolonged neuroplastic changes in nociceptive processes in the central nervous system (CNS). Furthermore, behavioural and psychosocial alterations may also take place (Sessle, 2009, p. 26).

Chronic pain reduces the quality of life, such as disturbances in appetite and libido, and can even lead to further psychological and emotional disturbances. It impacts on an individual's sleep patterns, social and family life, self-esteem, and motivation. Pain of this sort may consume the individual's life and they may feel "evicted" from their lives and their bodies (Gamsa, 1993; Flor, 2009; Sessle, 2009).

Psychological distress influenced X's physical state. Her chronic pain was not based on a biological illness; however, her psychological and emotional state was influencing her behaviour. Loss, rejection, and anger were so embedded in her emotional make-up that it would not allow her to progress beyond this pain.

X's identity seemed to relate to her desire to *have* fibromyalgia and if this was disputed, it was a blow to her existence. Her physical pain could be easily rectified and managed by a change in lifestyle; however, it was the mental suffering that she was not ready to give up. Perversion is not limited to a person's sexual behaviour, but may influence all of an individual's experiences, relations, and attitudes to reality. (Abel-Hirsch, 2006, p. 99). However, it is a means, in the form of a fetish, to a level of gratification and satisfaction.

There is a growing body of evidence that pain without an organic reason is based in the psychic mechanisms of the mind. Pain is a human phenomenon—a symptom or a manifestation of the modulations of the psychosignature created within the subject's psychomatrix. Experiences from birth (or earlier) are imprinted in the matrix of the unconscious mind creating a signature unique to the expressions of pain.

Why pain? We propose that pain is the first experience and therefore the first impression or imprint on the matrix. It is the primary emotion that one is born with from which all other emotions ensue. From birth, there on, the duality of the subject's existence is cemented and proceeds along the road of events and experiences that continue to impress upon the unconscious as well as the psychomatrix.

Pain that is "diagnosed" as chronic pain is an example of how what is repressed makes itself known, in the attempt to *deal* with the dynamics of one's multidimensional existence. The subject's relationship with his pain is manifested in his sense of existence and therefore impacts on his sense of identity.

Sufferers of chronic pain find themselves in a narcissistic space of isolation where the focus is on self-gratification which therefore, breeds a hyper-vigilance to and with *being in pain*. The search for the cure for chronic pain continues as some individuals go on to seek relief in self abusive behaviour such as, addictions and deprivation.

CHAPTER SIX

Addiction

Introduction

An addiction, I propose, is similar to the phantom limb and chronic pain syndrome as all three share the common threads of persistent and unremitting, physical, chronic pain, but, more significantly, emotional and psychological pain and suffering. They share the elements of fear of loss, annihilation and rejection, as well as the desire to escape, and the subject's need for reality to be concealed, such as within denial, in acts of self-preservation—be it perverse or other. These have been discussed in the previous chapters. Addiction, the focus of this chapter, is another such "syndrome". It has been theorised by some researchers that addiction can result in the repetitive use of a substance (or other compulsive behaviour) to ward off painful affective states, such as feelings of guilt, loss of self-esteem and loss of a sense of identity. Addiction can act to re-establish a central area of omnipotence and provides one with a sense of control of one's affective state. Therefore, addiction provides a sense of control and power that has been lost or taken away (Dodes, 1990, p. 400). It is functional within dysfunction. Hence, even though drugs are taken to achieve pleasure at first, subsequently they are used to ward off pain (Keller, 1992, p. 3).

This chapter will discuss this phenomenon of addiction and as with the other scenarios it is to evidence the subject's *relationship* to pain and its impact on his identity and existence. When we speak of "an addiction" the first thing that comes to mind is individuals who abuse illicit drugs/substances. This is not without good reason as the most commonly *seen* effects of addiction are from the results of drug taking behaviour. Addictions to other behaviours are not generally as obvious, for example playing video games, gambling, overeating, shopping, and sex, to name the most commonly advertised addictions.

The topic of addictions is a wide and complex topic with many layers of discussion. This chapter will not specifically focus on substance abuse or any specific addiction but the *primary element* that classifies a set of behaviours as an addiction, which is the compulsion to repeatedly engage in such activities to the point where it impairs the ability to form meaningful relationships as well as productive, effective, normal day-to-day functioning.

We need to take into consideration that there do exist individuals who indulge in certain kinds of such activities, in secret, living their lives, from an external perspective, quite "normally" functional.

Nevertheless, in order to discuss the subject-pain relationship within the phenomenon of addiction, it is essential for me to explore the most common components of addictions which have been generally discussed throughout research in this field. I have found that these fit into three main categories: biochemical/organic/genetic, behavioural and psychological. In doing so, I will also examine some of the theoretical explanations within each component. Each component is significant when discussing the topic of addiction however; my focus will be on the psychological component, and the rationale behind addictive behaviours. Here again will be my endeavour to evidence the subject-pain relationship and the role it plays within identity and existence.

It appears that the use of mind-altering substances has been part of every culture of the world. The theories of addiction take us from a need "to gain divine knowledge" (Loose, 2006) to more recent theories of addictions being a disease. The disease theory is heading the scientific research and according to research by the National Institute on Drug Abuse (NIDA, 2010), it is a comorbidity with diseases of the mind and therefore a "mental illness". Dr. Volkow, director of NIDA suggests:

We need to first recognize that drug addiction is a mental illness. It is a complex brain disease characterised by compulsive, at times uncontrollable drug craving, seeking, and use despite devastating consequences—behaviours that stem from drug-induced changes in brain structure and function. These changes occur in some of the same brain areas that are disrupted in other mental disorders, such as depression, anxiety, or schizophrenia.

Due to the complexities of the human condition, interactions of brain, mind, and body with internal and external environmental influences, none of the theories, of course, comprehensively explains addiction. Addiction has a complexity of components from within which any given combination has the possibility of creating the symptoms of repetitive, compulsive, self-destructive behaviour (NIDA, 2010, p. 1). This can also be said about the phantom limb and chronic pain syndromes.

Pleasure, it appears, is the reward that we desire. Freud proposed, referring to the *reality principle,* that the reality of it is that we must exercise a measure of responsibility. Nonetheless, the influences of our own biology, the environment and our own cognition and behaviour dictate how we actually respond to these desires. The question is then, when and or why does this "seeking" become pathological, as in addictions? As I have stated earlier, addiction is characterised by compulsive, at times uncontrollable (drug) craving, seeking, and use *despite devastating consequences.* Thus, it is pathological when the seeking of pleasure and reward is at the expense of physical, psychological and emotional health, human relationships, and is an effort to escape from unresolved, unconscious emotional trauma and other realities of life.

Bozarth (1994), further postulates that motivation can be either a desire for (appetitive) fulfilment/satisfaction, pleasure seeking, and behaviour directed toward goals such as sex and food; or an aversion to a condition that is unpleasant, such as pain:

> The notion that hedonic mechanisms might provide direction to behavior can be traced at least to the Greeks (e.g., Epicurus); Spencer (1880) formalized this notion into psychological theory and suggested that two fundamental forces governed motivation— pleasure and pain. Troland (1928) suggested that pleasure was associated with beneception, events that contributed to the survival of

the organism (or species) and thus 'benefited' the organism from an evolutionary biology perspective; pain was suggested to be associated with nociception, events that had undesirable consequences for the organism. (p. 5)

This speaks to the focus of Freud's work as well, who expressed a similar opinion about pleasure and pain; he also stated that both are necessary in order for one to fulfil desire. Knowing only pleasure or only pain, besides being impossible, would defeat the purpose of desire.

I will explore the psychoanalytic theories of the unconscious (underlying) and unresolved, emotional issues of pain that the subject strives to relieve or escape from by whatever means he can find. I will also examine the components of self-preservation, defence of affect (managing intolerable states) and self-regulation and elements of narcissism, neurosis, and perversion.

It will be evidenced that the subject's relationship with his pain is, at times, too overwhelming to manage in any other way accept to try to run away from it. However, in the process, pain is perpetuated and according to Loose (2011), "addiction is a choice for *Jouissance* that is administered independent of the structure that determines the social bond with other people" (p. 5). The desire for a *quick fix* waylays the need for developing human relationships, as well as long-term gains from creating an emotionally stable and productive life. The unbearable material from the past is repressed; however, as they press to the surface the pain of these emotional issues increases with every attempt at escape. I propose that behaviour, such as found in addiction, paralyses or even *amputates* part of the subject's sense of identity and meaning of existence. The phantom remains as it begs to be acknowledged within the chronicity of symptoms.

What is this compulsion to repetitive, destructive behaviour symptomatic of, or has it become the illness itself, such as the gangrenous leg that needs to be amputated or a fibromyalgia, without a specific cause, which becomes perpetuated within the lifestyle of the individual, who remains in denial? This begs the question, then, how does one "amputate" a behaviour or remove the "ache"? I propose that compulsive behaviour, such as an addiction, can only be managed if the root illness can be uncovered, treated, managed, and reconciled. Otherwise, the phantom of desire and denial continues to struggle to keep the lid on erupting, unresolved emotional trauma.

Definition of addiction

The most commonly found definition of addiction is that it is an uncontrollable compulsion to repeat a certain set of behaviours regardless of its negative consequences. Using drugs, or participating in certain types of behaviour, can precipitate a pattern of conditions recognised as addiction, which includes a craving for more of the drug or behaviour, increased physiological tolerance to exposure, and withdrawal symptoms in the absence of the stimulus. Most drugs and behaviours that directly provide either pleasure or relief from pain pose a risk of dependency.

Addictions, whether they are to substances or behaviours, share these characteristics:

> *denial*—an inability to realistically admit the negative consequences that result from the activity or substance; *compulsion*—an excessive preoccupation with seeking out or recovering from the substance or activity; *loss of control*—setting limits that you are unable to stick with. (NIDA, 2010)

Addictions can also be influenced by the opponent process reactions (Solomon, 1980). For example, the terror of jumping out of an airplane is rewarded with intense pleasure when the parachute opens. Because of opponent process, criminal behaviour, running, stealing, violence, acting, test-taking, gambling, and self-harm as in deprivation or drug taking, can become habit forming.

Addiction can be said to be a state of being enslaved to a habit or practice or to something that is psychologically and or physically habit-forming to such an extent that its cessation causes severe trauma.

Components and theories of addiction biochemical/ organic/genetic components

It is a well-known suspicion that the search for pleasure is one of the most fundamental reasons why individuals resort to drugs and substances of abuse. This is also one of the most influential reasons why some of those people become addicted. However, even when we speak of the neurobiological processes in the brain, we see that at first the drug achieves the pleasure. On the other side of the trip, though, it becomes a quest to escape the pain.

How the reward systems in the brain functions, when triggered by noxious substances, is the neurobiological processes that explain a factor in addiction. The brain produces the biochemical process that induces euphoria which also impacts on one's behavioural as well as psychological responses. Bozarth (1994) explains that there is:

> [A] biological mechanism mediating behavior motivated by events commonly associated with pleasure in humans. These events are termed "rewards" and are viewed as primary factors governing normal behavior. The subjective impact of rewards (e.g., pleasure) can be considered essential (e.g., Young, 1959) or irrelevant (e.g., Skinner, 1953) to their effect on behavior, but the motivational effect of rewards on behavior is universally acknowledged by experimental psychologists. (p. 5)

Research on genetics and the brain, conducted at the University of Utah, under the auspices of the National Institute on Drug Abuse (NIDA, 2006), has evidenced that addiction is a "chronic disease". This is based on findings that in fact drug use (and other compulsive, addictive behaviour) effects changes in the brain which results in a compulsive desire to use a drug or engage in repetitive high-risk behaviour. There are a number of factors, such as genetics, environment, and behaviour that influence an individual's risk of addiction, lending to the view that addiction is a complex disease. The research has shown that scientists usually look for biological differences that make an individual more or less vulnerable to addiction. There is no one particular "addiction gene" that has been discovered. However, there are a number of genetic values that influence this susceptibility in certain individuals. It is important to remember, though, that just because someone has a susceptibility to addiction does not mean that it is inevitable that he will have an addiction problem in their lives.

There is a possibility that an individual with a certain gene make-up is more (or less) vulnerable to an addiction, or experiences varying degrees of severity to withdrawal symptoms if they try to quit. On the other hand, there may be genetic factors that make it more difficult for someone to become addicted; for example, an individual may experience nausea from a drug that makes others feel good. Addiction is a complexity of factors and as Glen Hanson stated in a video presentation:

Scientists will never find just one single addiction gene. Susceptibility to addiction is the result of many interacting genes. Social and environmental factors contribute to this risk of addiction. It is becoming increasingly clear that genetic factors also weigh in. Like other behavioral diseases, addiction vulnerability is a very complex trait. Many factors determine the likelihood that someone will become an addict. (University of Utah, 2006)

Of all the people who experiment with drugs, research shows that roughly ten per cent become addicted. There is a combination of environmental and genetic factors that influence the likelihood of addiction. There are many elements within the environment, just as there are within the genetic make-up of an individual, which will impact on an individual's decision making process towards using drugs. There are environmental influences, such as family circumstances (divorce, conflict and abuse within the family) and whether or not a parent has a favourable attitude toward drug use. Other environmental factors are those of school and friends/peers, such as those who engage in anti-social behaviour and favour drug use. There is the community and its socioeconomic status, for example a community's attitude toward drug use, low neighbourhood attachment and community disorganisations, where there is nothing for kids to do after school, and no opportunities for young people to get involved in productive activities to learn to be part of their community.

All of these factors place a young person, as well as adults, at risk of addiction. The risk of addiction can develop in any of these environmental domains. Studies on the vulnerability to alcoholism for example, show that there is evidence that such genes are genetically transmitted, however it is not to discount that the environmental domains have their own set of influences. This is evidence to suggest that there is increased vulnerability due to biochemical changes caused by many substances of abuse (ibid.).

From a neurobiological perspective, drugs cause sudden and dramatic changes to the synapses in the brain. They bypass the five senses, smell, touch, sight, hearing and taste, and directly target and activate the brain's pleasure and reward centre (dopamine system) causing a dramatic and intense surge of pleasure. This places the brain in a compensatory process where it reduces the number of dopamine receptors at the synapse. Consequently, the action leaves an increase of the dopamine in the nucleus acumens which is what causes the surge of pleasure—a high. The uptake of the dopamine is hindered by the drug which occupies and fools the cells into releasing high levels of dopamine into the synapse where there is, consequently, a lack of uptake receptors.

As the effects of the drug wears off the individual needs more of the drug to achieve the same surge of pleasure or high. This is commonly known as "tolerance":

> As the brain continues to adapt to the presence of the drug, regions outside of the reward pathway are also affected. Brain regions responsible for judgment, learning and memory begin to physically change or become "hard-wired." Once this happens, drug-seeking behavior becomes driven by habit, almost reflex. This is how a drug user becomes transformed into a drug addict. (ibid.)

There are a variety of substances available that are used and abused for their effects as explained above. Each one behaves in a similar manner albeit in varying degrees. Keller (1992, p. 3) states: "[T]he addicted person is vulnerable not only to genetic influence, but also to many substances of abuse that cause biochemical changes resulting in habituation and physiological dependence, changes that are more or less powerful depending on the substance."

Research conducted by Bejerot (1980, pp. 246–255) suggests that addiction represents a newly acquired drive state arising from exposure to chemical substances that affect brain chemistry. The new drive state can overpower natural drive states such as hunger and sex.

Behavioural components

Environmental factors tend to have a significant impact on the risk of addiction, particularly in a predisposition of genetic factors. The *NIDA Research Monograph 30* has supported an extensive amount of research on the several theories and perspectives on addictions. Regarding this particular component, for example it cites a research study, *An Interactional Approach to Narcotic Addiction* conducted by Ausubel (1980, pp. 4–8). It evidences the influence of environmental factors that precipitate narcotic addiction. The study suggests two significant factors. One significant factor is the degree of access to the drugs. It explains, for example, that the risk of addiction to narcotics is higher in urban slums than in middle-class suburbs, due to the influence of economics and the family and community environment and attitudes toward behaviours, such as drug use. It also explains one of the reasons why drug addiction was virtually zero during World War II while normal commercial channels for illicit drug trade were disrupted. The article states:

> No matter how great the cultural attitudinal tolerance for addictive practices is, or how strong individual personality predispositions are, nobody can become addicted to narcotic drugs without access to them. Hence the logic of a law enforcement component in prevention. (p. 4)

The second and most important predisposing factor in the aetiology of narcotic addiction is the impact of prevailing degrees of attitudinal tolerance toward the practice in the individual's cultural, subculture, racial, ethnic, and social class milieu. This factor explains the various differences in incidence rates between lower and middle class groups, Europeans, Americans, and some Orientals as well as between members of the medical and allied health professions.)

> The crucial and determinative predisposing factor, which, therefore, constitutes the most acceptable basis for the nosological categorizing of narcotic addicts, is the possession of those idiosyncratic or developmental personality traits for which narcotic drugs have adjustive properties. Thus it is obvious that narcotic drugs are more addictive than, say, milk of magnesia, because their greater psychotropic effects have adjustive value for these personality traits. Chief among these effects is euphoria, which is highly adjustive for inadequate personalities, i.e., motivationally immature individuals lacking in such criteria of ego maturity as long-range goals, a sense of responsibility, self-reliance and initiative, volitional and executive independence, frustration tolerance, and the ability to defer the gratification of immediate hedonistic needs for the sake of achieving long-term goals. (Ausubel, 1980, pp. 4–5)

Thus, this is one example that there is a powerful behavioural component to the addiction syndrome. The behaviour can result from positive as well as negative reinforcement of that behaviour. The neurobiological processes are influential in perpetuating compulsive drug using behaviour; however, we cannot discount the significance of environmental factors. As I have discussed above, upon administration a drug bypasses all five senses and goes right to the brain affecting the reward centre (the dopamine system). The individual experiences a surge of intense pleasure (positive reinforcement), however during the period of "coming down" from this "high" the experience is the direct opposite of pleasure (negative reinforcement). There is an intense desire to repeat the experience. This behaviour is in response to the decrease in pleasure and increase in pain. Another point to consider, for the benefit of the discussions in the book regarding subject-pain relationship, is that the more intense the pain the more intense the desire for what is beyond the pleasure.

There are a variety of reasons for why an individual becomes involved in this type of behaviour; for example, this could be due to stress, childhood and other traumas and grief, anxiety, or depression. Any of these factors could be associated with different underlying psychopathology. There is a feeling of wellbeing, which is positive reinforcement for the behaviour which perpetuates the compulsive, repetitive behaviour. When an individual becomes so involved in the drug use that it is the only form of managing unfulfilled needs and wishes, it develops into an addiction. The negative consequences are feelings of guilt, loss of self-esteem and loss of identity, results in repetitive drug use to overcome these feelings—at first to achieve pleasure; however, it becomes a quest to escape the pain (Keller, 1992, p. 3).

Identifying types of drug/substance users would also identify the continuum of addiction or compulsive behaviour, around which society generally exists. Research has shown that users fall into certain categories, and as Wurmser (1974) has identified, there are, generally, three types of users of illicit drugs. This would also apply to those other behaviours, as mentioned above. On a continuum of use, the first category of users is the experimental or casual user who will use either out of curiosity, or to fulfil an initiation into a peer group, but does not feel the need for the consequential effects. The second is the recreational user whose aim is, basically, occasional or frequent intoxication. Within the third category falls the compulsive user who feels that the high provides him with *what is missing*, and is unable to give up the "high" regardless of the dangers and risks. Although it is, generally, the case that the casual or recreational drug user is the focus of attention in the media, perpetuating the vast amounts of wide speculations (pp. 822–823).

When considering the behavioural component of addictions one of the most significant domains in the environment to assess is the family. Within this domain, the considerations should be focused on the ongoing behaviour in the family context, changes and/or repetitive patterns during certain periods of time, and the interpersonal and contextual functions of drug abuse. Stanton (1980) states that symptoms of addiction occur within a context and serve certain functions within the context of the family domain not only for the drug user, but also for others in that environment (p. 147).

Families generally progress through similar developmental life stages, such as birth of first child, attending school, leaving home, death of parent/s or spouse and so on. Each one of these events is a "crisis point" as inevitable changes occur to progress development. However, these critical points, albeit at times difficult, are generally managed and got through. On the other hand there are those families who become "stuck" at a particular stage, and "like a broken record" they go through the same processes repetitively developing and perpetuating problems and unable to progress beyond the crisis.

This is applied to, and is significant especially within, families where patterns of compulsive drug-using behaviour are found. Research indicates that these families have experienced some kind of premature loss or separation during the family development cycle. There are correlations between drug addiction and immigration, or parent-child cultural disparity. There is evidence in research which indicates that the rate of addiction for offspring of people who immigrated either from another country or from a different section of the country was considerably higher than the rate for the immigrants themselves.

> It might be added that immigrant parents are also faced both with the "loss" of the family they left in their original culture and their own possible feelings of guilt or disloyalty for having deserted these other members. In any case, what appears to happen is that many immigrant parents tend to depend on their children for emotional and other kinds of support, clinging to them and becoming terrified when the off-springs reach adolescence and start to individuate with non-immigrant families of drug abusers, a high proportion show traumatic, untimely, or unexpected loss of a family

member, experiencing more such early deaths or tragic losses than would be actuarially expected [...]. This has led to the idea that the high rate of death, suicide, and self-destruction among addicts is actually a family phenomenon in which the addict's role is to die, or to come close to death, as part of the family's attempt to work through the trauma of the loss; in a sense, addicts are sacrificial and rather noble figures who martyr themselves for the sake of their families. (Stanton, 1980, pp. 147–149)

There is also the element of intense fear of loss and separation found among these families. There is a sense that the addict does not function effectively due to their high level of neediness, and dependence and lack of a sense of responsibility. However, closer observation of the whole family generally reveals that when addicts begin to succeed (in a career and/or in treatment or in other areas of their lives) they are in fact developing more autonomy and are moving away from this dependent pattern. At this point in time, it is almost inevitable that a crisis occurs in the family. Thus providing an environment for the addict to revert to some kind of failure behaviour, and the family problem dissipates.

> The implication is that not only does the addict fear separation from the family, but that the reverse is also true. It is an interdependent process in which failure serves a protective function of maintaining family closeness. The family's need for the addict is greater than or equal to the addict's need for them, and they cling to each other for confirmation or, perhaps, a sense of "completeness" or "worth". (ibid., p. 149)

The dynamics of the behavioural component within addiction are intriguing when viewed through the lens of this knowledge. In day-to-day evaluation and assessment of children and families, as a mental health clinician, although not restricted to but mostly from lower socio-economic status, I see evidence of these very roles and functions of the individual as well as the family. Many families come in with presenting issues of drug abuse. Further assessment reveals a high rate of domestic violence, sexual, physical, and emotional abuse within these families. A compelling piece of this puzzle is that research has also indicated that a high proportion of individuals who engage in compulsive, addictive behaviour, have been severely abused, sexually, physically, emotionally as children themselves or have siblings who were sexually abused. It can be concluded from these indications that these addicts are suffering from severe post-traumatic stress disorder to some degree and their addiction is a means to escape.

In the *NIDA Notes* publications, director Dr. Leshner (1998) comments on the ongoing research by NIDA (National Institute on Drug Abuse), stating that one of these efforts is the work of the research expert panel convened by NIDA in 1996:

> [The panel] reviewed the research on the role of childhood trauma in later drug abuse. Among the panel's conclusions was that the characteristics of the trauma, the child, and the child's environment interact to either buffer or aggravate the impact, which subsequently can produce a wide range of dysfunctional behaviours that can include drug abuse.

In another sphere of the behavioural component, I would like to explore another theory of addiction that is not far from Freud's (1920g) pleasure-pain, pain-pleasure, and the compulsion to repeat theory. Freud describes his theory of the pleasure-pain paradox in his investigations throughout his work. His investigations, no doubt, have provoked and propelled further research in all spheres of psychological processes in human behaviour, which subsequently has had its impact on many theories of addictive behaviour. Behavioural psychologists, for example, have taken this paradox one step further, in modern day psychology, to attempt to explain why so often actions to derive pleasures turn into compulsive addictive behaviour and, conversely, why our painful experiences can habitually lead to sustained feelings of pleasure and even happiness.

The opponent-process theory is one such theory that was developed by Richard Solomon in the 1970s. Solomon was a behavioural psychologist at the University of Pennsylvania. His theory at the time was not seemingly appreciated, however it was published in 1980 in the journal *American Psychologist* under the title "The Opponent-Process Theory of Acquired Motivation: The Cost of Pleasure and the Benefits of Pain", a paper that influenced the trajectory of certain research in the pleasure-pain paradox. In his paper, Solomon evidences his finding through experiments conducted on animals as well as human subjects. As Freud attempted in his 1895 *Project* (1950a) to map memory and motives of human behaviour, Solomon maps a sophisticated understanding of the physiology of the nervous system and, as Freud did, provides a framework of memory and motives to explain behaviours and emotional experiences in areas as diverse as addiction, thrill-seeking, love, job satisfaction, and cravings for food or exercise.

Solomon's theory is that we have pairs of emotions that act in opposing pairs, such as happiness and sadness, fear and relief, pleasure and pain. When one of these is experienced, the other is temporarily suppressed. This opposite emotion, however, is likely to re-emerge strongly and may curtail or interact with the initial emotion. Thus, activating one emotion also activates its opposite and they interact as a linked pair. To some extent, this can be used to explain drug use and other addictive behaviour, as the pleasure of the high is used to suppress the pain of withdrawal.

Sometimes these two conflicting emotions may be felt at the same time as the second emotion intrudes before the first emotion wanes. The result is a confusing combined experience of two emotions being felt at the same time that normally are mutually exclusive. Thus, we can feel happy-sad, scared-relieved, love-hate, and so on. This can be unpleasant but as an experiential thrill, it can also have a strangely enjoyable element and seems to be a basis of excitement (Solomon, 1980).

The framework suggests that the opponent-processes can be useful in adaptation and survival however, has the intoxicating potential to lead to compulsive, addictive, and destructive behaviour. Motives are based on the innate needs of the libido; however, Solomon's theory explains how new motives can be established due to repetitive stimulation of innate desires such as, hunger and sex. For example, consider a drug addict's situation: before addiction sets in, he experiences euphoria with use of the drug with a few painful consequences. However, as drug use continues he develops a tolerance to it that requires higher doses to acquire the same "high". At the same time, cravings and feeling of distress increase without the drug, leading to an increase in withdrawal symptoms, such as pain (as in opiate use, such as heroin) and drug seeking behaviour. Thus, the cycle of increasing drug use leading to addiction. The desire for food and sex therefore becomes secondary to the desire for drugs and the usual innate needs of the libido and self-preservation become paralysed.

Another example is of couples newly in love: following a period of initial infatuation (pleasure/euphoria) there is an experience of a

lowering of affection that leads to dissatisfaction, fights, and someth..
breakups. However, during reconciliation a renewed closeness is experienced for a period of time. It seems that the more intense the infatuation (pleasure/euphoria) the greater the pain (craving/desire) during
the period of *falling out*.

The behavioural component of addiction is, as we can see, influenced
by the actions of our neurobiology as well as the various dimensions of
our environment. The most significant influence, though, is of a psychological nature that involves our emotions and feelings and how we
view ourselves in relation to our internal and external environments.

Psychological components

Of course, all components of addiction involve the influence of the
emotional and psychological dimension. There are some intriguing
studies of medical patients who are exposed to narcotics as part of
their treatments. Psychologist Stanton Peels suggests that while these
patients build a physical dependence on the opioids, they are able
to protect themselves against addiction by thinking of themselves as
normal people with a temporary problem, rather than as addicts. He
opines that even though conditioning theories provide guidelines to
understanding addictive behaviour they are "limited by their ability to
convey the *meaning* the individual attaches to his behaviour and environment" (Peele, 1998).

It seems that the meaning one attaches to the object, such as pain (or
pleasure), is what makes a difference to his relationship with it and how
he uses it.

In his book *High Society: Mind-Altering Drugs in History and Culture,* Jay (2010) presents an example of another investigation into the
culture and history of drugs and how they have travelled, been used,
and evolved through time and societies. It indicates, as many other
researches have, that drugs are a significant element of the human race
which have a long cultural, political, and religious history of use for their
mind-altering characteristics. While giving a rendition of how various
societies present their use of their choice of mind altering substances, at
first glance, it paints a lazy romance of the "feelings" then weaves the
dichotomous picture of pain and pleasure. For example, he describes
the morning rush of people with their coffees, across cities in North
America, which is not too far different to the regular, desert pilgrimage

of the Huichol people of Mexico, who continue to harvest the peyote cactus for their rituals. And yet another "normal" daily scene, further along the south in Colombia and Brazil, where he describes the street children who intoxicate themselves sniffing or inhaling petrol-soaked cocaine residue and aerosol sprays (Jay, 2010, p. 1).

Throughout history, permeating through cultures and societies, there is the need for mind alteration whether it is the rush needed to ease the grind of a stressful job, the pathetic search for something to relieve boredom and hopelessness, or the pursuit of insight from a higher power. Humans seem to find it necessary to alter the psychological workings of their minds to give them the (emotional) courage (in their minds it is very real) to manage the dimensions of their lives that appear to lack power and control.

The fundamental element for us here is "mind-altering". Whenever "drugs" or drug abuse are spoken about it is in the context of mind-altering substances. Why do people want their minds to be altered? What is it that addicts people, not to drugs, but to their minds being altered? Drugs, of course, are the vehicles for this journey, without which the world would not have this *topic* to debate and analyse. When I think about this I realise that "mind-altering" is not so much speaking of the chemical alterations of the brain, but in fact it is the emotional context and dimension of the person which is in debate. This then, is more so, significant to my book as within this premise lies the issue of the subject-pain relationship.

Jay (2010), as others have done, explores the history of drugs, where they come from in the world, who used/uses them, the economic, political, and cultural conundrums, is it bad or good, legal or illegal, and the arguments that ensue, but, what of it? He investigates the subject's relationship with drugs or his drug of choice. I propose that it is not the subject's relationship with drug but instead it is a question of the subject's relationship with his pain.

Research, including that which has been discussed here, has indicated that severe anxiety, grief, trauma (including childhood abuse) and disasters and stress may be the cause of a high percentage of addictions. Trauma, biological and environmental, is the other piece of the addiction puzzle, along with the susceptibility of genetic transmission, and the effects of the drugs (or certain behaviours) themselves. Could we not conclude that an addiction may be, in fact, self-medication, an attempt at self-preservation, and a defence against feelings of annihilation?

All of this, which stems from the conglomerate of pain within the unconscious and a desire for the (lost) object, now presents as a need to *be in pain* in order to feel pleasure or what is beyond pain. The compulsive and repetitive nature of addictions is the perverse seeking to resolve the trauma and of that which is beyond the pleasure which is only more pain: pain that may ensue and that in turn could achieve a level of the pleasure pursued. It is a relentless cycle which perpetuates a desire for that which cannot be satiated. The subject's relationship with his pain is that of interminable desire contained within a narcissistic space.

As Wurmser (1974) proposes, compulsive drug use is a primary symptom of underlying disturbances, not the illness itself. In his paper, *Psychoanalytic Considerations of the Etiology of Compulsive Drug Use,* he describes the rationale for this proposal from observations of individuals whose drug of choice is removed. In these circumstances the individual would quickly replace that drug with others in order to achieve a similar objective—relief from depression, suicidal attempts, violence, and anxiety attacks etc., issues that were most likely present prior to the introduction of drugs. These symptoms would reappear with a vengeance when the subject is deprived of his drug of choice, throwing him into a desperate search for another drug to give him a similar relief. In these cases, it has been shown that withdrawal from the drug had little bearing on the success of treatment unless the psychological and emotional issues were addressed, (1974, pp. 822–823).

Throughout his writings, Freud (1895, 1916, 1909d, 1917, 1920g, 1926) discussed that the cause of the subject's pain is a response to the same, unconscious, unresolved emotional trauma. As has been discussed previously in this book, the unconscious hoards the pain of loss, abandonment, and rejection, provoking subjective responses, at varying degrees throughout one's developmental stages. This pain is at the root of an addiction which perpetuates unhealthy habits or rituals of compulsive behaviours that paralyses the progression to physical, emotional, and psychological wellbeing. What does this mean? Addiction is an obsession to a compulsive set of behaviours to achieve one outcome—pleasure at the expense of all else, even if it means creating more pain. If whatever is causing the pain is not addressed it perpetuates the pain by keeping the problem rooted in the unconscious, emotional dimensions of the mind.

Confronting the pain does not mean that it will evaporate into thin air and disappear. It means taking responsibility for one's actions and behaviours, and the consequences, which implicates not only one's self but also others. Pain, at a certain level, remains as part of the "hum" of reality. It is a part of one's conscious awareness as a distinctive qualitative experience. We can go so far as to say it derives its character from a combination of one or several conscious experiences such as emotions and sense of self. Chalmers (1997) says, "pain is a paradigm example of conscious experience" (p. 9).

However, in addiction the sense of self becomes imprisoned within the "self". The sense of self within the pain experience in addiction seems to reside within a space that is not allowed to transcend beyond the bounds of its desire. It has in effect given up its outward transcendence to an illusory self within. Loose (2006) postulates that:

> [A]ddiction is an independence of the Other. That means that if the relationship between the subject and the Other is one thing, addiction is something else (and somewhere else). In other words, symbolic castration and lack can be accepted (but repressed), disavowed or rejected (foreclosed) by the subject, but one way or another, addiction seeks administration. Anxiety and guilt are hidden at times, but paradoxically maintain an "obvious" (hidden) presence. (p. 217)

In being "something else" I propose that it is clear evidence of the relationship between the subject and his pain. Pain becomes the Other as it is objectified by the subject in his submission as he seeks to placate it with pleasure. I propose that when we are confronted with the symptoms of addiction we experience great fear as the repetitive compulsions instil a sense of profound loss. The subject's cry of anxiety turns toward the alienation of addiction. Pontalis (1981) explains the blurring of this boundary:

> … narcissistic cathexis following effraction—and now we are bordering on traumatism; or object cathexis following loss—and now we are bordering on mourning. Here again, too strict a division would not be pertinent, the very property of pain being to blur the frontiers. No doubt psychic pain depends—in the final analysis—on

object-loss, whether real or fantasmic—but to recognize the fact does not get us any further, for this loss is also the origin of anxiety … and of desire. In the case of pain, the object ceases to function as a possible surety; he is, at best, a substitute, and behind this substitute, there is always another one. Infinite "transference". Irremediably lost but eternally maintained, the object cannot be recovered through representation, which renders present another: the same yet different. Where there is pain, it is the absent, lost object that is present; it is the actual, present object that is absent. Consequently the pain of separation appears to be secondary to a naked, absolute pain. The psychic scene is populated only by shadows, the psychic *reality* is elsewhere, not so much repressed as encysted. (pp. 199–201)

From some psychoanalytic perspectives, substance abuse is considered a symptom associated with the oral or most primitive stage of development and represents an attempt to establish a need-gratifying symbiotic state. Addiction is also a result of impairments of the ego, and disturbances in the sense of self, involving difficulties with drive and affects defence, self-care/self-preservation, dependency, and need satisfaction (Dodes, 1990; Khantzian & Mack, 1983; Wurmser, 1974).

Khantzian and Mack (1983) take this a step further to add that the key desire is self-preservation. They explain that there are a set of complex functions that have been designated as "self-care", "self-protection", and "survival", and that the failure and impairments in the natural development of these ego functions explain a wide range of problematic human behaviours. They state that, although denial, conscious and unconscious self-destructiveness, psychological surrender, and other determinants can explain some human self-destructive behaviour and impulsivity:

> [W]e have been equally impressed that personality structure and character pathology of certain individuals leave them vulnerable and susceptible to various dangers that result in personal injury, ill-health, physical deterioration, and death. We believe such people are often not so much compelled or driven in their behaviour as they are impaired or deficient in self-care functions that are otherwise present in the more mature ego. (p. 209)

Here, again, it is evidenced that addiction is an interaction of more than just one component. There are several variables, even within the psychological component, that impact and influence an individual's character and personality, causing them to be susceptible to addictions—not least those of genetics and the environment.

The theory of self-care as a developed system of functions includes elements of libidinal investment in self-worth, care and protection of oneself, a capacity to anticipate danger and to respond to the cues, the ability to control impulses in the face of known, harmful consequences, satisfaction and pleasure in appropriately overcoming situations that present risk or danger, sense of self sufficiency and insight about one's external and internal environments, ability that is assertive or aggressive enough to protect oneself and developing skills in "object relations, especially the ability to choose others who ideally, will enhance one's protection, or at least will not jeopardize one's existence" (ibid., p. 210).

Considering the domain of the family and its stages of development, we see the most significant psychological influences. The ability for self-care and self-preservation is developed within the stages of development in relation to the family's development. Psychoanalytic research suggests that during the early stages of development children depend on external objects for self-preservation and could at the same time experience real threats to their "survival as a result of external dangers, injury, insult, and aggression" (ibid., p. 212).

This research further indicates that the instinct of self-preservation is present early in development than has been supposed. It indicates that small children manifest early concerns about death and self-preservation. The capacity for self-preservation begins earlier in human development and the importance of quality and quantity of nurturance and care in the earliest phases of mother–infant relationship has been stressed by researchers such as Winnicott (1953, 1960) and Mahler (1968), cited in Khantzian and Mack (1983, pp. 212–214).

Within the structural theory of the mind, Freud (1913j) formulated the fundamental functions of the ego. Self-preservation was a part of the ego instincts and he referred to these as instincts which serve the "preservation of the individual" not those which "serve the survival of the species" (p. 182). He explained, initially, that within narcissism the ego instincts are non-libidinal aspects of narcissism, however he ultimately rejected this view in favour of the perspective that self-preservation is itself erotic in a narcissistic sense stating that "the instinct of self-preservation is certainly of an erotic kind, but it must nevertheless have an aggressiveness at its disposal if it is to fulfil its purpose" (Freud, 1933b, p. 209).

Khantzian and Mack (1983) considered the perspective that addictive behaviour serves as an attempt at (aggressive) mastery over poorly understood and passively experienced suffering, in an attempt at self-preservation. A failure in, particularly, maternal nurturing can leave certain individuals "ill-equipped to maintain and regulate" their self-regard and self-esteem because of impairments in ego-ideal formations. This leads further into the element of narcissism in addiction (p. 214).

Dodes (1990) states that addicts have a sense of profound powerlessness, which betrays a specific narcissistic impairment. Addiction in this instance strives to restore or re-establish a sense of power and is correspondingly, impelled by narcissistic rage. "This rage gives to addiction some of its clinical properties" (p. 397). He states:

> [I]n light of the core narcissistic importance of maintaining psychic control, it is significant that drugs are a device par excellence of altering, through one's intentional control, one's affective state. [...] addictive behavior may serve to restore a sense of control when there is a perception that control or power has been lost or taken away. (p. 400)

The neurotic part of all of this is that addictive behaviour is in itself inherently a matter of being out of control, a paradox of ego functioning as well as loss of elements of ego functioning (ibid., p. 401). This "being out of control" betrays underlying problems and is a means to deflect from facing those problems—a desire for the gratification or satisfaction of needs and on the other hand a desire to escape the pain of this desire.

I suggest that throughout Freud's work it is quite clear that he pursued a wide perspective of knowledge to uncover the roots of the individual's psychological and emotional pain which influence his behaviour. Beginning with his discussions in his *Project* (1950a) of the body/brain's neuronal system and chemical activity, and throughout his subsequent work in psychoanalysis, all roads led to pleasure but first to desire (pain). It is apparent, in investigating Freud's work, that he was eluding to the influences of the neurobiological, behavioural, and psychological domains that impact on human behaviour. Self-preservation, it seems, is a fundamental element in psychosocial development that impacts one's sense of self and the meaning and worth of his existence. This process begins in infancy during the primary narcissistic stage that is essential to future development of ego functioning.

It seems clear that his endeavours were to pin point the relationship that the subject has with his pain. His attempt to master his pain is an attempt at maintaining a sense of self-preservation. Freud (1920g) presents an example, to evidence his theory, in a game (Fort/Da) of repetition. He explains that the compulsion to repeat is an effort, on the subject's part, to gain mastery over his pain by re-creating the experience repeatedly. It is not the actual event, but a metaphor that symbolises the content of the event, such as the loss of a loved one, so as to create an emotional response (satisfaction/pleasure) within the state of pain. Once the pain is gained, another action is then taken to satisfy that pain in order to gain pleasure. The little boy throws the spool that is tied to a string away from him, out of sight (loss/pain) then, reels it back to re-find it (pleasure). The little boy is in control of losing as well as finding the object in recreating the occasion of his mother leaving, a distressing moment, and then returning, a pleasurable moment. However, he does not have any control on when she leaves and when she returns—no power or control to choose or demand otherwise. Hence, the process of the game is in order for him to feel in control (pp. 14–17).

The key in this, I propose, is that there are some things that are beyond one's control. However, in some subjects this is an unacceptable notion (failure of development of ego functioning during early stages), creating a susceptibility to a compulsion to repeat, such as in addiction, in order to create an illusion of complete control. The state of ultimate equilibrium and satisfaction is the cessation of one's existence (and all pain) in death. Most people, we assume, do not wish death upon themselves. However, what they do wish for is to experience an emotional space (in their minds) that brings them as close to that equilibrium as possible.

I could make an assumption that in this game the little boy's relationship with his pain (loss) is that of master and slave. Pain initially is the master as it makes the subject feel out of control. The subject is then in control as he re-enacts the pain experience to gain control/pleasure and master pain. However, pain continues to overshadow the situation, as the subject is not in control of every element of his situation. On the other hand, pain is a necessary motivator to achieve pleasure (ibid.).

Another suggestion in response to this assumption is that, perhaps, the subject's relationship to his pain is co-dependence, which expresses itself in a desire to be controlled by something other than oneself, within the confines of compulsive behaviour. The subject attempts to relate to his pain through such mediums, as the "chronic pain syndrome" or the "phantom pain syndrome", as well as "the addiction syndrome".

The emotional state of the mind is influenced by biochemical changes induced by repetitive use of drugs, however it can also be altered by repetition of certain cognitive processes (catastrophic thinking and attitude towards a particular problem or issue) and behaviours, such as gambling or playing video games. These may create a co-dependent process in the mind. With regards to this co-dependence, it has been evidenced to indicate that in cases of "catastrophising" subjects, there has actually been alteration in the neuronal and brain chemical activity. For example, in a case of chronic pain, Haythornthwaite (2009) has investigated how (among other factors) "catastrophising" in patients with chronic pain alters neuronal activity and states to perpetuate the pain. She states:

> [P]ain related catastrophizing comprises a set of negative emotional and cognitive responses to pain that include helplessness, magnification of pain, and rumination. [...] Pain-related catastrophizing appears to amplify central nervous system processing of noxious input via alterations in spinal and cortical modulatory systems. (pp. 271–280)

As far as changes in the processes of the brain which are further influenced by cognitive and psychological processes, Ramachandran, as previously discussed in this book, has investigated the brain's ability to compensate for missing limbs due to "remapping", and states that "the brain abounds with maps":

> These maps are largely stable throughout life, thus helping to ensure that perception is usually accurate and reliable. But [...] they are also being constantly updated and refined in response to vagaries of sensory input. (1999, p. 40)

In a co-dependent relationship to pain we can see the impact of certain kinds of catastrophic thinking within the realms of feelings of helplessness and powerlessness. As we have seen, addiction alters the neurobiological as well as the emotional processes of the brain and mind, setting the process of cognition and behaviours on an altered trajectory. The addict will do anything to alleviate the pain and to achieve pleasure. Therefore, he will do anything to master pain in order to keep it as close to him as he can for he knows only too well that the (repetitive) release from pain will gain him pleasure. As Keller has suggested, drugs may be taken, initially, to achieve pleasure however consequently they are used to ward off pain (1992, p. 3).

In the grips of addiction, we can see that there is a need for pain to *resolve* another pain. Is pain a sort of a defence mechanism such as Freud's theory of "conversion"? "[I]n hysteria, the incompatible idea is rendered innocuous by its *sum of excitation* being *transformed into something somatic*. For this I should like to propose the name *conversion*." (1894a, p. 49)

Freud further states:

> [T]he excitation which is forced into a wrong channel (into somatic innervations) now and then finds its way back to the idea from which it has been detached, and it then compels the subject either to work over the idea associatively or to get rid of it in hysterical attacks—as we see in the familiar contrast between attacks and chronic symptoms. (ibid., p. 50)

Apart from the neuronal changes in the brain, there is another element that changes, the emotions and the processes in the mind. Therefore, the idea of "mind-altering" in the context of addictions is significant. This thesis suggests that this very element is a fundamental concern within addictions and consequently the subject's relationship to pain.

According to Freud (1894a), conversion disorder is where unacceptable emotional instincts and desires are converted to physical symptoms. And as expressed by Ford and Folks (1985) conversion is where unconscious drives, such as sexuality, aggression and dependency, that have been prohibited internally, find expression in physical symptoms. Physical symptoms allow for the expression of the forbidden wish or urge but also disguise it. Other psychoanalytic explanations focus on the need to suffer, or identification with a lost object (Ford & Folks, 1985).

An event triggers the prohibited and repressed emotional instinct that threatens to invade the conscious and destroy the ego's control.

The ego allows the repressed to make itself known by the increase in excitation; however to relieve the unbearable impact on the conscious emotions it allows the process of conversion. In so doing the subject is able to gain control of his suffering. It is easier to say that he has a physical pain than to say that he has a psychical pain. The (physical) pain can thus be controlled freely, and for that moment, side steps the threat of reliving a past emotional trauma. In addiction mental and emotional pain are transferred to the experience of the whole body giving the impression of the body lost in the experience of pleasure, oblivious to all else.

The state of intoxication creates a space in consciousness that is *medicated*, so as not to feel the pain of the whole impact of what is repressed. The effect is the conscious being split between feelings of euphoria as well as the physical, physiological reactions of the body. The high and euphoria from the administration of the drug fulfils the prohibited, repressed emotional desire for the lost object without having to actually depend on the other to fulfil its desire (Loose, 2001).

Freud (1894a) postulated that repression or "intentional forgetting" leads to pathological reactions such as hysteria, obsessions, or hallucinatory psychosis, and are bound up with the splitting of the consciousness. The ego is split between decreasing the emotional potency of the "incompatible idea" of what has been impressed in the memory, and converting this energy to the somatic sphere (pp. 48–49).

Therefore, even though, a symptom of physical suffering has been created the *phantom*, of the prohibited emotional and unresolved instinct or desire, remains in the conscious mind. Freud (1894a) explains:

> [I]f someone with a disposition [to neurosis] lacks the aptitude for conversion, but if, nevertheless, in order to fend off an incompatible idea, he sets about separating its affect, then *that effect is obliged to remain in the psychical sphere.* The idea, now weakened, is still left in consciousness, separated from all association. *But its affect, which has become free, attaches itself to other ideas which are not in themselves incompatible; and thanks to this 'false connection', those ideas turn into obsessional ideas.* (pp. 51–52)

The "obsessional ideas" are the defence of the ego against threats of the repressed. The ego resists making connections with the repressed material. If, in analysis, this resistance is removed, it is important to keep in mind that the repressions remain, still, to be undone and worked through. The compulsion to repeat certain behaviours, to continue to gain control over the resistance of the unconscious, "repressed instinctual processes", is ever present (Freud, 1926, pp. 158–160).

As Pontalis (1981) expresses:

> Where there is pain, it is the absent, lost object that is present; it is the actual, present object that is absent. Consequently the pain of separation appears to be secondary to a naked, absolute pain. The psychic scene is populated only by shadows, the psychic *reality* is elsewhere, not so much repressed as encysted. (pp. 199–201)

The compulsion to repeat certain behaviours is to relieve that part of the conscious that is split, but remains in the psychic sphere. Since the symptom causes some kind of incapacity, the ego appears to, in some way take revenge, by what Freud (1926) calls a "gain from illness" (pp. 98–99). For example, in the case of some alcoholics and drug abusers (from the point of view of it being an incapacitating disease), they are unable to find employment due to the restrictions of their chronic "illness". This is similar to Freud's example of the war veteran who had got his leg shot off in the war so that he did not have to work any more, (ibid.). He goes on to state that it is "very rare that the physical process of 'healing' round a foreign body follows such a course as this" (ibid.). It is here that there is an idea of Freud's opinion around the successful treatment of addiction within the process of psychoanalysis.

This process of the ego places it within a "narcissistic" space as it fulfils its need for appreciation and self-preservation. The ego accepts the symptom instead of allowing the repressed material to the surface. The ego puts up its resistance in a "gain from illness", as if there is nothing that can be done to relieve the symptom, but it does not fool the superego into the same illusion. The superego has its own resistance "that seems to originate from the sense of guilt or the need for punishment; and it opposes every move towards success" (ibid., p. 160).

Between the two there is the id that demands attention in its "compulsion to repeat" behaviours, as in repetitive drug use, to gain or regain control, satisfaction and pleasure by re-enacting the event that triggered the behaviour in the first place.

The experience of helplessness or powerlessness, are central factors for addicts. The treatment that Alcoholics Anonymous offers within their twelve-step recovery programme focuses on these factors. The focus of the first step of recovery states: "we admitted we were power-less over alcohol" (Dodes, 1990, p. 4).

I can conclude, therefore, that although there is merit in exploring the many types of mind-altering drugs available on the various international markets, how they react in the body and the brain and what they do to the mind and the need of the conscious mind to keep repressed, prohibited, emotions at bay, it is also imperative to explore the correlations within the processes of mind-alteration. These would be in conjunction with the contributions of the external environment and genetics as well as behavioural and psychological factors.

The processes in the mind that are active in repression are altered by drug addiction and/or repetitive, compulsive behaviours. Loose (2006) suggests that "Freud was opening up the possibility [...] that addiction and masturbation, as pleasure producing activities, could be related to mental pain as the cause of these activities" (p. 33). However, he speaks in the context of the subject's relationship to drugs. The compulsion to repeat, as in the case of an addiction which is a symptom, is a "substitute satisfaction".

Loose (2006) explains:

> Freud began to realise that the hysterical symptoms contain an element of pleasure. This made him think that the first traumatic scenes might perhaps have been somewhat pleasurable for the infant. Freud had stumbled upon the elements of infantile sexuality. The infant must have experienced a conflict between the pain of trauma and something pleasurable. (ibid.)

I would like to speculate here that, on another level, it is the pain that the subject relates to which is the primary addiction. Pain is the object of desire, and in the attempts to prevent the pain or ease the pain, pleasure ensues. When the pleasure (high) wears off, the move is then to avoid pain. However, without the pain there would not be the need to seek pleasure. Freud states, "pain occurs in the first place [...]. The transition from physical pain to mental pain corresponds to a change from narcissistic cathexis to object cathexis" (1926, p. 171).

The object that has been created by the subject then, is pain to which inevitably he lives in relation to. His behaviour, therefore it follows, is contingent upon this relationship.

Addiction: a neurosis

Neuroses, generally, comes about from the frustrations of basic instincts. These are situations where the ego's effort to repress its instinctive desires has failed. The subject suffering neurosis is one whose ego has lost the capacity to allocate his libido in some way. The demands of what is repressed and the failure of the ego's capacity creates a symptom that has the potential to be worse than the original conflict that it is trying to replace. The symptom allows the ego to waylay the conflict between ego and id and that allows him to experience pleasure; however, it is in a way one which is often debilitating.

Neurosis can be caused by either internal emotional impulses not properly repressed by the ego, manifesting in other ways, or external traumatic experiences such as childhood traumas, usually of a sexual nature. However, it is usually a combination of the two that will manifest in a neurosis.

A neurosis, then, looks like a symptom or a set of symptoms that betray unresolved, unconscious emotional trauma. This is experienced by an individual as psychic pain—pain that was experienced in earlier life, and which he has not been able to process or work through, consciously. The repression that resulted was an unconscious process as a defence against the unbearable emotions and there is, possibly, no conscious memory of the event or occurrence. The nature of the past traumas could be of a variety of incidents that could be perceived as traumatic incidents. There is usually no conscious recollection of the event. However, instead the subject will develop nervous symptoms which are experienced as an illness or disorder. The symptoms could be those of drug abuse among others, such as eating disorders, self-harm, anxiety, depression, and sexual problems.

I would conclude that a neurosis is the formation of behavioural or psychosomatic symptoms as a result of the return of the repressed. According to Freud, there are those cases in which the solution of a conflict by a neurosis is harmless and tolerable, socially. He argued that even healthy life mingles with certain trivial and unimportant "symptoms". He went on to say that the neurotic who needs treatment simply has more debilitating symptom-formations that prevent enjoyment and active achievement in life (Freud, 1905, 1916, 1926, 1930a).

Freud (1905) did make a connection between neurosis and addiction:

[I]t must suffice us to hold firmly to what is essential in this view of the sexual processes: the assumption that substances of a peculiar kind arise from the sexual metabolism. For this apparently arbitrary supposition is supported by a fact which has received little attention but deserves the closest consideration. The neurosis, which can be derived only from disturbances of sexual life, show the greatest clinical similarity to the phenomenon of intoxication and abstinence that arise from the habitual use of toxic, pleasure-producing substances (alkaloids). (pp. 215–216)

It seems that here he is alluding to the process of compulsive use of drugs which lead to the achievement of pleasure, initially; however this then turns into attempts to ward off pain. This in turn leads to consequences of the subject's disconnection from his external environment, as he is preoccupied with the compulsive behaviour of acquisition and administration of drugs. Freud, I suggest, is comparing this to actual neurosis where the subject is preoccupied with warding off painful, repressed material and "disturbances" of earlier sexual development.

Freud (1930a) expressed that trauma caused by relationships to others are the biggest threat and barrier to people's achievement of happiness. Thus isolating oneself from social interactions with others can be one way of solving the problem. On the other hand, this produces another problem. In avoiding others, one also avoids social connection and fulfilment. An alternative would be to resort to something that will achieve a similar satisfaction. However, this pleasure has a short life and quickly brings on the negative and opposite affects that perpetuates addictions. Initially the drug use is to achieve pleasure and consequently to avoid pain. In this way addiction compares to neurosis in that it manifests in symptoms to defend against the pain of repressed, past trauma (p. 78).

Perversion in addiction: a degree of self-preservation

When speaking of perversions in the context of this book I should clarify that it is the *perversion mechanism* that is the consideration and not the *disorder*. As such, we propose that addiction (or self-destructive, repetitive compulsive behaviour) is a perversion mechanism. Although, having said that, it would appear that, individuals caught up in a lifestyle of addictions (and other self-harming, self-abusive behaviour) present with symptoms that may very well represent a diagnosis of a disorder. As Stoller (2003) points out, as with neurotic mechanisms, so perversion mechanisms serve to preserve sexual gratification against childhood intrapsychic trauma and conflict. He states:

> Either way, since the original sexual impulse must be thwarted, disguised, and reinvented and the whole process perpetuated, since anxiety and risk-taking, violence, and revenge are hidden in the symptomatology, one must use a word that connotes this intense dynamic tension. (p. 111)

Addiction seems to be a complex, symptomatic manifestation of fear of loss, rejection and abandonment, anger, hostility, humility and a desire for escape and revenge. It affects, not only the individual, but also all others who come in contact with him or her. The need for self-preservation gone terribly wrong, it seems as if the subject is lost in a void that separates desire and self. The subject endeavours to maintain a separation by an object that he has created, and maintains, by his entering into the realms of addiction—destructive, repetitive, compulsive drug use (or other such behaviours). Kahn (1979) states that, "the pervert puts an impersonal object between his desire and his accomplice. This object can be a stereotype fantasy, a gadget or a pornographic image. All three alienate the pervert from himself, as alas from the object of his desire" (p. 9).

The addict uses the drug to reach the high that gives him the illusion of satisfaction and power over the object.

Addiction is an obsession with pain. Pain gives the subject a sense of having a "meaning" to his existence, however it is not without a sense of a desire for revenge upon the object of his desire, which perpetuates itself within compulsive behaviour. It is an angry admission that the object cannot be re-found in its original form, to avenge himself by gaining the satisfaction (as he reaches a "high"), and that the only way to achieve the ultimate equilibrium is to get back to the place before existence—death. He cannot have the object of his desire, and he cannot move beyond his desire in order to achieve success. Since the object is inaccessible the subject creates an allusion to it by re-enacting the "original" pain that was created by the conflict, during the infantile stages of development. Stoller (1986) states:

Freud did not believe that trauma caused perversion of sexual development until it caused conflict; conflict is awareness of the need to choose between alternatives and requires a development advanced enough that memory, judgment, and perhaps fantasy are beginning to influence behaviour. (p. 34)

The conflicts that arose during the libidinal developmental stages are the causes of the subject's perversions. These perversions, consequently, arose as a defence against unbearable emotional and intrapsychic conflicts. Freud believed that perversion in males was due to the fear of castration due to his desire for his mother. Castration would make the boy anatomically inferior and the same as a girl. In females, he believed that perversion was the result of her lack of ability to accept that she is already castrated resulting in her overemphasis on the value of her clitoris. This, in turn, prevents her from shifting to the more feminine vagina or makes her unwilling to turn to her father, in other words to heterosexuality, and therefore she fails to enter into the oedipal conflict as a feminine person who wants a baby—to replace the penis. She renounces her identification with her mother in this manner. "Perversion may mark failure at any step in the process of this oedipal [interpersonal] theory" (ibid., p. 35).

The elements of hostility, aggression, and revenge that are manifested in risk taking behaviours come into play in the perversion mechanism of addiction due to its unique relationship with loss, rejection, annihilation and identification. "The risk that one will again fully experience the early childhood trauma is the primary one that energizes perversion formation" (ibid., p. 115). For some people this is more terrifying than risking death or being arrested. Risk is part of the manifest content of the perverse act, as in masochistic (or sadistic), and is inherent in the dynamics of revenge. This brings to mind a statement that Loose (2007) makes, referring to an article by Rado:

Drugs provide a kind of satisfaction that by-passes the erotogenic zones. [...] Addiction, so to speak, sexualizes the whole body, providing it with, what Rado called, an "alimentary orgasm". What turns people into addicts is the predominance of an oral satisfaction that can be produced at will has all the hallmarks of an orgasm invading the body. (p. 103)

This brings in the consideration of the desire for control of the "object" that stands for the "object of desire", the external object. The subject will control the pain and the pleasure, and he has at his disposal his own body to achieve this. As Stoller (2003) stated, perversion is the erotic form of hatred.

The original trauma can be enacted within a fantasy to achieve an outcome of "triumph"—as in an act of revenge. However, there is a thin line between fantasy and reality. In addiction the fantasy becomes a reality in that the pestilence is put upon the subject's own body as if to purge the body of its desire and to avenge feelings of hatred, rejection and humiliation. The subject's own body becomes the object. The challenge is in the need to destroy the object as well as to achieve triumph over it by taking what is desired. Here, again, we see pleasure and pain become accomplices it the quest for satisfaction. There is also an element of omnipotence in the act of the addict as there is a sense that he can achieve all his desires without the other, therefore rejecting the object as he was rejected. Loose (2007), not too far off from Stoller's (1991) ideas, indicates that addiction is a search for sexual satisfaction that belongs to the stages of early infantile development. Hence, the addict's avoidance of normal sexual relationships. He goes on to say:

> Addicts are fixated to a form of satisfaction that belongs to the oral perversion that provides the direct satisfaction on an unconscious infantile drive that, for some reason, was never properly overcome or sublimated; so drugs and alcohol can function as substitutes for the gratification of infantile sexual wishes. (2007, p. 101)

One of the essential characteristics of addicts, he suggests, is their inability to deal with frustrations and demand immediate gratification. They satisfy this demand for immediate pleasure, through their compulsive use of drugs. It is significant to note his reference to the research by others who have identified connections "with narcissism, depression, mania, and paranoia" (ibid., p. 101). It speaks to the complexity of addictions as it implicates the neurobiological but, most significantly the psychosocial systems of the subject.

The "compulsion to repeat" is a narcissistic endeavour toward self-preservation at the expense of all else. It is a narcissistic seeking to fulfil the self's desire for pleasure from the mastery of the past emotional pain caused by loss, rejection, fear, anger. This can become a lifelong endeavour. Drug taking, and self-abusive behaviour, share similar patterns found in chronic pain sufferers. Pain is needed to perpetuate more pain/desire to gain pleasure. Somewhere in the unconscious of the individual lies the imprint of traumatic events and experiences that have the potential to awaken emotions that are painful and unbearable. Somewhere in the unconscious lurks the possibility of an emotional illness, whether drugs, or other behaviours/activities, are introduced or not. Addiction is a manifest symptom of this disturbance, on the one hand, and on the other hand, it is the disturbance.

As Loose (2002) has stated:

> [Freud] had discovered fantasy, infantile sexuality, the structuring effect of the Oedipus complex and the importance of language for an understanding of the psyche. Above all, he had discovered that human suffering was not caused in the first place by a clearly locatable external trauma but by a disturbing element within the psychic economy of the subject which ex-ists like an unprocessed remainder. Neurotics are no longer innocent victims of an external cause; something disturbs them from within. (p. 30)

In more recent studies it is evidenced that trauma can be repeated on many levels, such as, emotional, physiologic and behavioural, causing a variety of individual as well as social suffering. Anger can be directed at the self or at others. This is a key problem in people who have experienced a violation of some kind. This aggression is in itself a repetition of past traumatic events. Trauma occurs when external and internal resources are lacking or inadequate. This brings us back to discussions about the importance of nurturing, during the infantile stages of developmental, where a failure of this can leave individuals ill-equipped to maintain and regulate self-care and self-esteem. The implications for the development of the ability to care for oneself, as in self-preservation, during the initial stages of infantile development are crucial. A failure at these key stages sets the functional environment up for a variety of anxieties and the possibility of destructive, repetitive, compulsive behaviours (Khantzian & Mack, 1983, pp. 209–214).

A compulsion to repeat, as in addiction, is an unconscious desire to overcome trauma or to master the traumatic event and takes us back to infantile stages of development. No matter how we view this compulsion it appears to be an aggression upon the self, as we see from our discussions already. On the other hand, it is a desire to gain control of one's self and is an effort at self—preservation. It is a perverse need to take revenge, according to Stoller (2003), on the primary object (the mother). However, there is also an element of a desire to punish the self for being deficient, without adequate resources for protection from trauma in the first place. Within the complexities of unconscious emotions and unconscious guilt, addiction, as in other chronic pain, is evidence of a desire for revenge on the object, on the one hand and guilt and the need for punishing the self, on the other hand.

It is clearer today than ever before that the subject's life is influenced by suffering through the powerful forces of nature (natural disasters such as the Tsunami), his own weaknesses and feebleness of his own body (old age, incurable diseases such as cancer and schizophrenia), and the complex dynamics of relationships within the family and society (attachment, loss, poverty, war and terrorism, abuse). As regards the first two, Freud (1930a) further explains that we will never completely master nature, and our bodily organism, that is itself a part of that nature and will always remain a transient structure with limitations. Instead of this being a negative element, it actually presents a positive element to life as it not only makes us aware of our human limitations but gives us clues regarding our capacity. He states, "If we cannot remove all suffering, we can remove some, and we can mitigate some" (p. 86). Regarding the third point on the social source of suffering he stated:

> [O]ur attitude is a different one. We do not admit it at all; we cannot see why the regulations made by ourselves should not, on the contrary, be a protection and a benefit for every one of us. And yet, when we consider how unsuccessful we have been in precisely this field of prevention of suffering, a suspicion may lie behind—this time a piece of our own psychical constitution. (Freud, 1930a, p. 86)

Could it be that pain is the object which we desire? Addiction appears to be such a phenomenon. It is clear evidence of how unsuccessful we have been in precisely this field of prevention of suffering. And for the reason, namely, that addiction is "something" (or a lack of something) "in our own psychical constitution". There is a barrier that prevents the problem of addiction to be fully addressed and therefore, resolved.

Addiction ties the physical and the psychological processes in a relentless bind. When examining the state of addiction the question of whether or not drug use, or a "compulsion" to repeatedly engage in mind altering and, possibly, mind and body destroying behaviour, has any physical influence or is it at all psychological, arises time and again. Studies have shown that even though there is an element of physical influence, it is certainly less significant than the psychological and emotional elements of compulsive behaviour. The body becomes a sort of a *holding cell* for the desire of fulfilment, and its preservation becomes secondary to the preservation of desire and achieving pleasure. The body endures the pain for the sake of gaining satisfaction/pleasure. Therefore, addiction "inevitably ... very often" induces "a physiological dependence" (Wurmser, 1974, p. 823).

Freud's (1920g) determination to seek out the workings of the human being, and his desire to find balance, took him to his concept of the *pleasure principle* and *beyond the pleasure principle*. Freud's will to pleasure was dictated throughout his work as well as his own personal experiences. It brings into the conscious realm, to some degree, his desire to *use* his addiction, and pain, to inspire him ever onward in the quest to boldly excavate the complex and contradictory realms of sexuality and the unconscious:

> Freud observed on his own person that cocaine could paralyze some disturbing element and thus release his full normal vitality. He [...] was puzzled why in other people it led to addiction [...]. His conclusion was right, that they had within them some morbid element of which he was free, although it was many years before he was able to determine what precisely that was. (Byck, 1974, pp. 201–202).
>
> It was psychoanalysis that several decades later brought the first insight into the nature of addiction and its complex relationship to the effect of the drugs. In 1885, when Freud met the problem, he thought of the hunger for stimuli, of mental weakness, of lack of self-control as the decisive factors. (ibid., p. 347)

Loose expresses that Freud's relationship with cocaine was a "symptom" (2002, p. 11), and we propose that his addiction was a manifestation of his relationship with his (psychic) pain. What is significant, in his work toward uncovering and relieving psychic pain, is that psychoanalysis, as with other therapies, is not a cure for pain, but a reminder that we have pain due to (the various theories of causes), most significantly, loss and rejection—unresolved emotional trauma and a need for satisfaction and a sense of fulfilment and self-preservation.

Similar to the symptom of neurosis, addiction shuts out the unconscious, acting as a repression. However, the cost of this is high. Eagle (1998) states:

> Freud made clear his observation and belief that repression both exacted a cost and bestowed certain benefits. Thus, early on, he writes that banishing an unwanted mental content from consciousness both frees the ego from "incompatibilities,"—a benefit,—and produces hysterical conversion symptoms—a cost. Furthermore, in his later writings, Freud (1916–1917) also refers to the work of repression,—"a persistent expenditure of force" (p. 151),—and suggests that repression entails continual psychic effort and exacts a cost on the personality. (p. 88)

The paradox of addiction is that while it can act as a protective shield against the feelings of a loss of control over one's unconscious emotions—restoring a sense of control—it is also behaviour of being out of control that engages a self-destruct button. "Simultaneously, then addiction reflects both ego functioning and a loss of elements of ego functioning" (Dodes, 1990, p. 401).

The addiction of deprivation

Addiction is similar to other diseases, such as those that affect the heart and the brain. They disrupt the normal, healthy functioning of the underlying organs and if left untreated, can become a lifetime of terrible pain and at times have tragic consequences. On the positive side is the fact that these diseases are preventable and treatable (NIDA, 2010).

According to Marrazzi and Luby (1986), eating disorders are similar to an addiction. In fact it has been identified that anorexia may represent a profound psychiatric disorder that may give rise to an addiction to deprivation. This is the topic I will discuss in this section.

It is significant to consider the interaction between the neurobiological system and the psychological system when we speak about pain being relieved by another pain, for example psychological pain relieved by conversion to a physiological pain. However, a further serious correlation is when the neurological system of the body takes over the psychological systems in order to compensate for deprivation and therefore switching to survival mode. This is particularly seen in research that has been conducted with patients suffering from anorexia nervosa.

It seems that the initial stages of anorexia are certainly compelled by deep seated psychological and emotional trauma in early development. However, the later stages are perpetuated by the neurobiology of the body adjusting its processes to compensate for the state of deprivation, as will be explained further on in this section (Marrazzi & Luby, 1986).

In exploring various scenarios where destructive, repetitive, compulsive behaviour is found, it seems that the complexities of one's internal and external environments have implications which impact the ego functioning of an individual. In most cases of addiction we have come across unrelenting influences of past psychological trauma caused by, for instance, childhood sexual abuse, domestic violence (physical, psychological, and emotional), and other dysfunctional family and/or community dynamics, war, terrorism, poverty—to name only a few.

I would like to examine an example of childhood sexual abuse, as the prevalence of these cases, in my own work, seems to be on an increase. It comes clear, on one level, how perversion mechanisms, such as an addiction to pain through behaviours of self-abuse, can set in when the subject is faced with intrapsychic trauma and conflict, during the early stages of development. This is a unique case with a vast array of complexities, the most significant being that the subject is a nun who lives in a cloistered convent. Sister Marie Thérèse of the Cross (2008) suffered childhood sexual abuse from the age of two to eleven, at the hands of her grandfather.

First of all, it is of significance to note Anna Freud's (1981) summation of ego-psychological perspectives on incest expressing how molestation (childhood sexual abuse) disrupts the normal developmental stages of childhood sexuality and prevents the overcoming of the Oedipus complex and the subsequent transition to latency:

> Far from existing as a phantasy, incest is thus also a fact [...]. Where the chances of harming a child's normal developmental growth are concerned, it ranks higher than abandonment, neglect, physical maltreatment or any other form of abuse. It would be a fatal mistake to underestimate either the importance or the frequency of its actual occurrence. (p. 34)

It is also important to make note that the following is *my* analysis and assumption about the details of this case. I will look at some of the key elements from a psychoanalytical perspective that the manifestations of self destructive, repetitive, compulsive behaviour are a form of addiction, following the destruction of ego functioning in early development. Anorexia is a complex illness, particularly when there are issues of childhood sexual abuse (it is not exclusive to this as childhood damage, from other forms of abuse and trauma, are equally as significant, in many cases of anorexia). For the sake of brevity, I would like to look at only a few of the key factors, in order to evidence my assumption that this is a form of a perverse mechanism as found in addiction. The case is mainly significant in evidencing the level of impact the individual's relationship with pain has on their existence and identity.

Sister Marie is of White Irish ethnicity and was born in London. She is a Carmelite nun whose given name is Sheila. At the time of my interviews with her, she was fifty-six years old. She chose the name Marie Thérèse of the Cross upon accepting her vows into the cloistered order of the Sisters of Carmel. Sister Marie had been abused by her grandfather from the age of two up until the age of eleven (the year during which he died). She was devastated when he died, and hated him for leaving her with her "broken body". She hated him but at the same time, she loved him because after all she was "his little girl" and they shared a special secret. She stated:

> Although I was grateful I did not have to face the horrors of the abuse, I felt desperately alone with the consequences of it. Grandad had betrayed my love and trust, leaving me with a body I was ashamed to own. It seemed to be all my own fault. [...] he had made me promise not to tell anyone—still I was so afraid lest anyone found out. [...] I hated myself for being granddad's little girl and I cried it all deep inside. (2008, pp. 15–16)

The development of her sense of self-preservation had not only been interrupted but intruded upon. Sister Marie realised very quickly that this was a secret that could never be told and the reason, the tremendous emotional trauma of intrusion upon her body, was buried deep within her. She hated her grandfather for leaving her with a broken body that she could not appreciate and share with any other person, as it was now unworthy of love. She was humiliated and ashamed and at eleven years old, words made themselves available for her to formulate the tragedy of her experiences, which she was left with. She felt that the only way that she could protect herself now was to destroy the "bad little girl inside" so that she could be free.

Sister Marie recounts that she had realised at around the same age of eleven that she had a desire to "devote herself to the church". She encountered moments of realisation that confirmed to her that her dream was to become a nun and that she wanted to enter into the cloistered Carmelite order. One of these moments was when she saw one of the nuns from the convent walk across the street—in her long brown habit. She knew that she wanted to go away to the convent—to a place that she never had to leave. It was then that her struggle, and attempts to escape, began. She did not believe that she was worthy of becoming a nun, however she had decided that she would do whatever she had to, to make herself worthy. Sister Marie's account in her book, *The Silent Struggle*, details this very struggle with her "vocation" and her tremendous struggle with her deeply buried secret and her anorexia that on the one hand protected her from her memories, and on the other hand punished her for them: "I hated my body and did not want to eat anything that was good for it. I would never be good enough to become any sort of nun so I would have to die if I wanted to go to God" (2008, p. 25).

Sister Marie's ailment began with binging and purging that eventually worked its way to anorexia nervosa. According to Lacanian theory, this state of anorexia-bulimia could be understood more effectively from the perspective of *Jouissance*. The behaviour calls into view the theory of *beyond the pleasure principle* and the *reality principle*. "It is a very fine and delicate elaboration of the dynamic between anxiety and the Demand of the Other that can serve as a compass in this field" (Aguirre, 2011, p. 180).

Placing severe restrictions on her food intake was clearly taking control of the traumatic events in her past. She felt that it was her fault that the abuse continued because she loved her grandfather and this somehow made her "evil". She wanted to punish the "little girl" for her terrible sin and so placed grave restrictions on her obtaining "comfort". Sister Marie believed that in order to gain the reward of "Heaven" she needed to be rid of her "broken body" and was seemingly on the road to chronic suicide. In speaking about destructive behaviour in addiction, Khantzian and Mack (1983) stated that Freud's theory of a death instinct could best account for the "varied and manifold forms of human self-destructiveness, such as asceticism, martyrdom [...]. He considered such problems as forms of 'chronic suicide'" (p. 211).

Shortly after her grandfather died, Sister Marie began suffering with symptoms of an eating disorder that quickly worked into a full blown anorexia. Here she recounts the details of binging and purging, including taking laxatives, and inducing vomiting. Soon she would eat very little, restricting her food intake to the bare minimum, but then purge herself by vomiting and the use of laxatives. Her body began to deteriorate and she went from one extreme to the other—to the point of near death—as the organs within her body began to deteriorate. From the outside, she looked as if her body could not support any of its functions. Which concurs with Aguirre's (2011, p. 178) suggestion that "[T]here is that quality of the mortification of the body which is often encountered in the clinic of anorexia."

Neuroscientific research conducted by Margules (1979) is cited by Marrazzi and Luby (1986) to explain that the fuel created by blood glucose is critical to brain function and activity. Therefore, during starvation the neurobiological systems switch to survival mode to protect the brain from glucose deficiency by maintaining the blood glucose level at the expense of other organs (p. 196).

In one of my interviews with Sister Marie, she stated that anorexia was her "friend". It knew her secret so deeply that she felt as if she had to be true to it, this friend, who took care of her. She saw her life through this *relationship* with her anorexia—her pain. This pain embodied her life that consisted of her experiences of sexual abuse at the hands of her grandfather from the age of two to eleven. This is where she "lived" every day trying to figure out how to "destroy" the little girl who had had these experiences, trying to control this period of her life as she was powerless to do at the time. Anorexia gave her the control that she needed. It made her deprive that "bad little girl" who had allowed her grandfather to sexually abuse her.

She let him do that to her and, then, still loved him and missed him after he died. She stated that when she vomited or took laxatives that helped her purge her body and made her feel good. So much so that she wanted, actually needed, to do this to herself every time she felt the pain of her past. Anorexia let her objectify her pain and allowed her to distance herself from it. She separated the little girl who had been abused and who represented the terrible pain in her life, from her *self*. The pain thus became an external entity that she could control and manipulate. This way she also justified her punishment of herself. She stated that she needed anorexia to protect her from what had happened in her past, but she knew that it was also destroying her.

Sister Marie said that being in the treatment centre had taught her to understand her past trauma, her feelings, and her behaviour. Over time, this had helped her to manage her anorexia. However, one thing that she realised is that her obsessive preoccupation with destroying herself through deprivation was like an addiction, except that instead of indulging your body with drugs to get a high you deprive it of sustenance and abuse it. Every time she vomited, she felt relief, a sense of satisfaction that was a sort of a high as it relieved her pain. Research has evidenced that during starvation or food deprivation the body compensates by producing opioids to protect itself from the "pangs" of hunger. According to Marrazzi and Luby (1986) opioids are released and mobilised during states of prolonged deprivation. They hypothesise that this could be an underlying cause for an "auto-addictive process" for a relentless chronic anorexia nervosa (p. 191).

The deprivation gave her a sense of control over her past circumstances. She needed that sense of power and control over her life in the present so as to have the courage to be able to purge herself from any sin in order to be worthy of being a nun—she was determined to be a nun but more importantly, she wanted to be a cloistered nun. Sister Marie realised her dream of entering the Carmelite order, however not without great sacrifice as she struggled within the grips which the disease of anorexia had on her, physically and psychologically.

From a young age, she "befriended Jesus" and turned to him for comfort. She looked to him to forgive her so that she could remain in her dream—at the convent as a nun—devoted to her calling. Her sense of martyrdom was indestructible as she sacrificed her own body bit by bit in order to be worthy of her vocation to God—as she felt that she had been chosen for a life of poverty, chastity and obedience—to Him. In this way, her suffering held meaning for her and helped her on her mission to become a nun and to work as a nurse in the infirmary.

Her anorexia became worse, as the years progressed, and she had to succumb to going into a residential treatment centre—threatened by the fear that she would have to leave the convent if she did not. After a long, difficult struggle in treatment, she finally began to learn how to manage her anorexic illness. Here she had to disclose and face her past.

At this time, she was faced with her reality—that she hated the little girl inside of her, who was abused by her grandfather, and wanted to destroy her. Her anorexia became her accomplice in her mission to destroy this damaged little girl. From the age of eleven to fifty-six Sister Marie inflicted abuse upon herself to separate her *self* from her desire that was a complexity of emotional pain. This was a kind of "chronic suicide" that accounted for her tendency for anger and aggression that was manifested in her self-destructive behaviour.

Anorexia is a neurosis, in that it betrayed childhood sexual trauma. However, it goes beyond that. It is the subject's intense hatred of (her) self, the guilt and shame of her past experiences that can never be overcome. The symptoms of anorexia were a set of compulsive behaviours repeatedly unleashed upon the body. This seemed to be in an effort to separate the "little girl" with the secret and an already "broken body", and the person whose desire was to take revenge and to regain control of her helplessness and her powerlessness. Her desire to be a nun gave her a sense of omnipotence and magical thinking, as if by being in the realm of "God", she had a champion. Being a nun would put her in this realm of power. She secretly believed that if she could only destroy this bad little girl the good person would emerge.

From a neurobiological perspective, research evidences that once the body's survival system is mobilised past a certain level, anorexia becomes a lifelong battle. The reasons why an individual sets upon this route are complex. It has been shown that the beginning stages are no doubt psychological, for example, a sense of unworthiness and dissatisfaction with body image due to a multidimensional complexity of causes. However, as the behaviours continue the illness develops into a chemical disorder. It seems that there is not only a psychopathology of anorexia nervosa but, also, a pathophysiology. Psychodynamic concepts, such as psychoanalysis suffice to explain the initial and acute stages of anorexia; however, they fail to explain its chronicity and the nature of its resistance to treatment and sometimes fatal prognosis (Marrazzi & Luby, 1986, p. 200).

The neurobiology of anorexia nervosa is significant, then, and has been evidenced to explain the chemical reaction and changes within the body that could perpetuate the illness. However, the psychological bases of the dysfunction remain primarily significant. The psychological and emotional trauma that impacts the subject's intrapsychic processes is what triggers the behaviour. Therefore, treatment rests in the effective management of emotional pain. The question of what does success mean within a treatment programme has been debated, as it has been when considering other addiction treatments. The general paradigm is shifting to allow for how well one manages this (chronic pain) illness (Marrazzi & Luby, 1986).

In the case of Sister Marie, there was clear evidence in her book, *The Silent Struggle* (2008), as well as during our discussions, that her emotional pain was great yet that she had gained a certain power over it. On the other hand, she continues to battle with the damage that her behaviour, due to anorexia, has caused to her body. To see the impact and transition of how the illness can become a lifelong struggle one needs to consider the stages that anorexia can travel through. She explained how the anorexia has caused her reproductive organs to fail as her body had ceased to create the hormones that were needed. This further complicated the normal functioning of other organs in her body. She talked about what she had learned during her treatment and continues to learn, and her desire to share this knowledge with others who may be suffering similar pain.

Marrazzi and Luby (1986) have found that during prolonged deprivation of nutrition the body begins to alter its functions in order to conserve bodily resources, in the first stage of the illness. It then proceeds to alter its functions further by beginning to decrease the metabolic rate of the system and, hence, the metabolic needs of the body. In the advanced stages, it further alters its functions to reduce "species survival functions, which are not necessary to the preservation of individual organisms. These homeostatic adjustments, together with opiate analgesia and inhibition of sympathetic arousal, seem to represent a broad adaptation to the stress of starvation" (p. 195).

In further examination of the psychoanalytical concepts of anorexia, it appears that the development of ego functioning toward self-care, self-protection, and survival had been interrupted in Sister Marie's early developmental years. The violation of the sexual abuse by her grandfather destroyed her sense of safety and left her vulnerable. Sister Marie felt that the cloistered convent would be a "sanctuary" that would create an inner sense of safety. She was preoccupied with this thought daily, on the one hand, while she performed the self-harm, on the other, as she fought her sense of shame, guilt, and punishment. She was preoccupied with her desire for her grandfather as well as her hatred of him. In doing so she abused her body, it seems, in the same way that her grandfather did. The pain that she felt from her deteriorating body was the pain that she felt while being sexually abused. However, the pain of her actions also released a sense of "wellbeing" and control unlike when she was young, while her grandfather abused her. She wanted to be loved by her grandfather but did not know, at the time, how to protect herself from what he was doing. Even though she did not know, at the present time, how to protect herself from her own self-destructive behaviour, it was this behaviour that was also a defence and protection from those traumatic memories and emotions. She inflicted herself with pain, however the pain then provoked pleasure that perpetuated the desire for pain and so the cycle goes on.

At one point during her treatment, Sister Marie said that she was "heartbroken". At the time, she had begun to understand her illness and one way of doing this was to address "Sheila". This was her given name and the name of that "broken little girl" inside. She was afraid that she would never find Sister Marie Therese again. "Now, I had to accept the little girl I so wanted to disappear." She could no longer hide inside her habit feeling she had no right to be there (2008, p. 215).

Anorexia may also be viewed as a perverse mechanism, which is an attempt through destructive, repetitive, compulsive behaviours, to preserve sexual gratification against trauma. It consists of the subject's pursuit of gratification through hostility and vengeance, mystery, and danger that surround the traumatic attachment to the mother (Cooper, 1991, p. 20).

Perversion as such, in other words, is "sin". The idea of sin presents a sense of risk taking as in the pursuit of forbidden pleasures. The elements of guilt to compensate this then turns to punishment and a sense of vengeance and hostility directed toward the self but, then it becomes apparent that it is directed toward the mother. Stoller (1991) states that with sin, "the excitement comes from an awareness—conscious or unconscious—that one is harming, needs to harm, wants to harm. More precisely, the harm done is an act of humiliating in revenge for one's having been humiliated" (p. 37).

Sister Marie relates that before her grandfather came to live with them (she was two years old) she felt that she was always in the way and was beaten if she cried and her father was always "yelling" at her. Her mother seemed to be relieved when she could leave her in her grandfather's care. Her grandfather seemed to want to take care of her and seemed to be the only one that loved her (2008, pp. 10–12).

She even felt at the time that her father would be jealous since she was now her grandfather's little girl.

The first time that her grandfather did something to hurt her (she was four years old) she yelled out loud from the pain and her mother ran upstairs to see what had happened. Her grandfather said something to her mother who then proceeded to beat her. She felt at that moment abandoned, rejected, and humiliated. The pain of the humiliation was so much worse. Later her grandfather threatened her saying, "you ever make that noise again you will get worse" (ibid., p. 12). Her mother had abandoned her and failed to protect her, and she would carry it with her, in spite of her treatment successes. She depended on her mother's help, yet she wished to be away from her. She punished her own body as if punishing her mother for humiliating her, as if wishing her past experiences on her mother.

By the time Sister Marie began the process of her treatment for anorexia, in the residential unit at Springfield Hospital, her mother had died. Her mother had been giving her all the attention that she desired, and she felt that she was special to her. However, this was a double-edged sword with one side a "triumph" and the other side guilt and a need for punishment. She was determined, more than ever, to remain in the convent, and recalled her mother's distress at her interest in such a career. She learned to manage her anorexia enough to be able to return to the convent during and following her treatment phases.

Sister Marie's internal conflict lay in a trauma inflicted upon her by someone in her external environment. It was an act that was inflicted upon the child from the outside thus, rendering her powerless. As a child, and as is natural for a child, she was completely dependent on the adults around her for protection and a sense of wellbeing. The abuse was an intruder upon this sense of safety and self-preservation creating within her a sense of confusion and loss of control (Joyce, 1995).

Similar to the destructive, repetitive, compulsive behaviours of addiction, there is in self-abuse, as in anorexia, the aspect of superego pathology, where the faulty ideal formation is underlined. In addictions, the archaic forms of shame and guilt and the very primitive and global fears of humiliation and revenge play a dominant role in the social interactions of these patients. It appears that the aim of these destructive behaviours is to gain an affect that increases a sense of self-esteem, and control and the "re-creation of a regressive narcissistic state of self-satisfaction" is consistent. These behaviours are particularly evident during a "narcissistic crisis" that would entail a particular intense disappointment in others, in oneself, or in both—"so intense because of the exaggerated hopes, and so malignant because of its history's reaching back to very early times". Such crises are usually found in family crises coinciding during stages of maturation and adolescence (Wurmser, 1974, pp. 838–839).

It was at the beginning of adolescence, age eleven, when Sister Marie's grandfather died that her struggle with anorexia began. There were many other struggles that her family were going through yet, she had become preoccupied with herself. Everything Sister Marie achieved, from participating in family responsibilities to gaining entry into the convent seemed to be through the haze of her anorexia. Her constant battle was how, when and where she could do what she needed to do to fulfil her desire to maintain her body in the dilapidated state that it was—protecting herself from her guilt and shame.

She wanted to enter the cloister so that she would never have to interact with "normal society" again lest it re-victimise her. She had lost all trust in her environment and social relationships. She was so afraid of being powerless in the face of her past experiences. Her struggle continues with anorexic tendencies within her daily life yet, she is learning how to control the anorexia as she had allowed anorexia to control her.

Sister Marie's destructive behaviour served to ward off a sense of helplessness and powerlessness through the control she exerted over her body in order to control the pain that her memories gave her. She created pain through her behaviour in order to separate her from her desire—for the lost object. This drive, as in addiction, to re-establish a sense of power corresponds to the subject's sense of powerlessness and is "impelled by narcissistic rage" (Dodes, 1990, p. 397).

According to Stoller, perversion is a result of mixtures of three key unconscious fantasies constructed in the perverse defence against fears of passivity when confronted with rejection, loss and abandonment from the maternal object. At the basis of the subject's behaviour is the fantasy that gives him a sense of control and power. Within these fantasies are efforts to deny the experience of being the helpless and needy infant that is at the mercy of a frustrating and cruel mother.

> They erase passivity by denying human maternal control of oneself as human, by defensively converting active to passive, and by extracting pleasure out of being controlled. [...] Regardless of

whether sexual pleasure is consciously an aspect of the activity and regardless of the prominence of the fetish object, the perversion dynamic is in action whenever the body is treated as not human and mixtures of these three fantasies are present. (1991, pp. 24–25)

From this perspective the destructive, repetitive and compulsive behaviours of addiction—addiction to drugs or other types of self-harm—have elements of perversion as the body is used as a vehicle for revenge and defence against infantile emotional trauma, violation and conflict.

The concept of "unconscious guilt" and an "unconscious need for punishment" has the greatest influence on the initiation of self-abuse, as in drug use, as well as in relapse and relapse prevention. One of the theories of addiction by Kohut (1971), cited in Dodes (1990), discusses that addictive behaviour is seen as a gratification of instinctual needs or a reunion with a "forgiving parental object or an activation of 'all-good' self and object images". Kohut referred to addictions as "narcissistic behaviour disorders. [...] disturbances in addicts as due to the mother's failure to function as an adequate idealised self-object, and saw drugs serving not as a substitute for loved or loving objects, or for a relationship with them, but as a replacement for a defect in the psychological structure". Wurmser (1974) also emphasised a "narcissistic crisis" in drug abusers, in which the collapse of a grandiose self or an idealised object leads to feelings for which drug use is an attempted response: "an archaic overvaluation of the self or of others [leads to] the abysmal sense of frustration and let-down if these hopes are shattered [...] and thus to the addictive search" (p. 400).

The most important elements in addictions and other self-harming behaviour, such as within the complexities of anorexia, are the roles of power, helplessness and rage and consequently the role that these behaviours play in managing the sense of loss of omnipotence over one's own affective state. It is clear that the loss of control over one's emotions and feelings is highlighted by the loss of this control in psychic or mental trauma. The sense of helplessness is imposed on the ego and it is overwhelmed by an instinctual drive (affect) which it cannot manage without excessive anxiety. This sense of powerlessness and helplessness is what amounts to "psychic trauma". "The ability to be powerful over oneself and one's internal state may also be described as an inherent aspect of narcissism" (Dodes, 1990, p. 400). He further explains that according to Spruiell (1975, p. 590) narcissism is "the pleasure in efficient mental functioning [...] the regulation of mood [...] and [...] a sense of inner safety and reliability" (ibid.).

I have seen in cases of addiction, as well as in other cases of self-abuse, the role of these behaviours is an attempts to achieve this "efficient mental functioning" and to restore a sense of control. The addict will use drugs and an anorexic will starve herself or vomit or take laxatives to purge herself of painful desires to achieve a sense of inner safety and reliability. These individuals covet their feelings and have a need to possesses them, not wishing to expose them to the world—there are his feelings (of pain) alone to enjoy (or despise), in the privacy of his mind. The excitement of the risk of these behaviours, and doing something that is outside of the constrictions of conformity, or committing a "sin", first of all, add to pleasures sought by these individuals who are involved in addictive, self-harming behaviours. And second, it adds to the complex issues of treatment.

What is verbalised by the individual is rarely the exact truth; in an effort to keep this pleasure and pain hidden, lest it be taken away and they lose the device for self-preservation and gratification. The need for this is to fill the emptiness and lack of wholeness and lack of control. As Sister Marie stated, if she gave up anorexia she would have admitted defeat and lost the last remnants of her sense of control over her past. The need for control is clear, as discussed earlier. Even in the middle of an assessment or treatment the individual will continue to *hide* behind words and behaviour, that she thinks will protect her and her activities. The issue of building a trustful relationship with another is one of the essential elements within any such treatment even before treatment can begin.

As I have been discussing, addiction seems to be tied intimately to an individual's attempt to cope with his internal emotional and external social and physical environment. It is a result of severe ego impairments and disturbances in the sense of self, involving difficulties with drive and affect defence, self-care, dependency, and need for satisfaction.

Mental pain, as has been discussed, stems from loss—namely loss during the infantile stage of development—of the primary object, the mother, the breast, and the fulfilment of primary desire. Freud (1905) indicated that addiction can be related to a fixation in the oral stage of libidinal development and, by implication, he hinted at a possible connection between addiction and perversion (p. 182).

[T]he avoidance of the so-called normal sexual encounter with the Other indicates the search for a sexual satisfaction that belongs to an earlier stage of infantile sexual development. Addicts are fixated to a form of satisfaction that belongs to the oral stage of sexual development, with addiction being a kind of oral perversion that provides the direct satisfaction of an unconscious infantile drive that, for some reason, was never properly overcome or sublimated; so drugs and alcohol can function as substitutes for the gratification of infantile sexual wishes. (ibid., p. 101)

There is a desire to cover up this deficiency and compensate for it with the repeated use of substances and other forms of self-abuse. I have learned as well that there is pathology present within the narcissistic sense of self. Disruptions and disturbances in a person's early development, particularly around infantile stages, where there is the highest dependence on being nurtured, are the roots of the breakdown. Here there is found to be a narcissistic vulnerability and overcompensation for self-preservation. Drugs are used, in this case, as a compensation for this lack.

Defences are set up in order to contain the unconscious longings and aspirations of the individual. It is because of this disavowal and "massive repression of these needs that such individuals feel cut off, hollow and empty [and that the] addict's inability to acknowledge and pursue actively their needs to be admired, and to love and be loved, leave them vulnerable to reversion to narcotics" (Khantzian, 1978, p. 196).

Sister Marie's (Sheila's) case is unique compared to other cases of self-harm and addiction as such, in that in examining the details one is rather cautious about the elements of the unconscious desires of ones sexuality. Nuns are a holy community who dedicate their lives to God, taking vows of chastity, poverty, and obedience. Albeit Sister Marie was a nun who was dedicated to her work, she was also a woman who had experienced not just sexual relations, but a sexual relationship of childhood abuse and violation. The struggle for her was twofold. First, it was an effort to live up to her commitments and vows. In order to do so she felt that she must get rid of her previous life and what she had learnt about human sexual relationships, through the acts of abuse, which she was a victim of.

Second, I propose that her guilt for feeling a desire for not just her grandfather's love, but for desiring him sexually, was what drove her to punishing her*self*. The perverse, repetitive behaviour, which she was committed to in an addictive process, was a defence against her guilt, which she had reconciled to, as being insurmountable struggle and her cross to bear and the pain which she desired in order to gain the ultimate pleasure that she called heaven. Her relationship with pain was such that it was the toll she had to pay for the passage to being worthy of her calling.

The case of B

This second case study will also be examined from a framework of the psychoanalytical theories discussed in this chapter. We will consider Wurmser's (1974) theory that the specific reason for the onset of compulsive drug use lies in an "acute crisis" in which the underlying narcissistic conflicts are mobilised and the affects connected with these conflicts break in with overwhelming force and cannot be coped with without the help of an artificial "affect defense" (p. 838).

I could also apply some of Khantzian and Mack's (1983) theory of self-preservation and self-care where they describe these as a set of ego functions, and suggest that failures and impairments in the development of these functions can explain a range of troubled human behaviour (p. 209). Dodes' (1990) theory of addiction being a set of behaviours that serves to ward of a sense of helplessness or powerlessness via controlling and regulating ones affective state, can be particularly relevant to the following case (p. 397).

Addiction, being an aspect of the dimensions of human existence, presents a highly complex set of behaviours. It is impacted and influenced by any number of variations of physical, psychological, and biological elements. It is important to keep in mind that there is a spectrum of drug use. On the one end there are those who are the occasional and recreational users and on the other end are those whose mental suffering is so intense that it manifests in a pathological compulsion to repetitive, relentless drug use.

Considering the challenges of its complexity, I acknowledge that this is an ongoing battle to know what really works best. It is also important to note that many an addict has come out "clean", and has changed his life around, on their own without any particular addiction/mental health intervention. To say here that *the war* on drugs is a rather useless exercise, is to stress the point that it should really be *the quest* for treating emotional pain as in mental suffering and not a war on drugs (Peele, 1998).

This topic of addiction is also significant to my argument as it further illustrates the subject's relationship with pain.

Throughout the treatment sessions with B, I identified three major needs, which were: (1) his need to feel safe and to survive; (2) his need to preserve his emotional state, and to feel in control over his life; to overcome his intense fear of annihilation, to find meaning in his existence and pain; and (3) a need to be compensated for loss, rejection, abandonment, and humiliation. He desired to fulfil his sense of loss and longing and to regain a sense of omnipotence (as in power and control) over his environment that had caused him his suffering. The complexities lay in the subject's experiences in his early childhood and his progression through life up to the present.

I was one of the mental health/addictions therapists at the treatment centre where B presented, and where we offered assessments and person-centred analysis and therapy to our clients. This case was of interest to me due to his unique presentation, as well as his progression through his process of change, mostly, due to his own convictions and working closely with strategies that he created for himself. He relapsed a number of times, yet every time he came out he was even more determined to get to the goal that he had set himself. It was as if he needed to master his pain and use it to his benefit.

This example shall address some of the factors that may have caused the phase of addiction which this individual experienced. His addiction seems to have been due to a sense of loss during his earlier stages of development and his endeavour to (re)find the "object" that would satisfy this loss. He experienced feelings of being out of control, a lack of identity, humiliation, and meaninglessness in his life. This resulted in feelings of emptiness, of a vacuum within which he experienced phases of unrelenting desire for satisfaction and fulfilment—humiliation, anger, guilt, a need for revenge and a sense that he deserved to feel good.

Presenting symptoms

B presented with concerns regarding depression and anxiety and feelings of hopelessness. He confirmed the use of various substances, but no indication of suicidal ideation at that time. He was in his early twenties, of mixed Latin/European ethnicity, and an only child. In the initial interview, B stated that he did not think he needed any help; he knew what he had to do to deal with his problems, and had only come in to the clinic on the insistence of his doctor.

As the sessions progressed, B expressed a fear of having a heart attack (a fear of dying) due to his periodic experiences of tachycardia (racing heart beat), and sleeplessness. Medical examinations, by his doctor, ruled out any irregularities in his physical health. Therefore, it came down to the fact (as he admitted) that he was using drugs on a regular basis, and experienced severe withdrawal symptoms including, nausea, tachycardia, headaches, irritability and anxiety attacks.

B was an articulate and pleasant young man with a good sense of humour and laughed easily, even at himself. However, he also tended to giggle, even during serious discussions, as if there was a need to hide from his problems. He expressed his shame and guilt around his drug use and, initially, appeared impatient with the questions that were put to him. However, gradually he seemed comfortable enough to relate his story. It seems that B's bursts of giggling were an effort to waylay some of the anxiety that he experienced when in the sessions.

This particular aspect of B's presentation seemed significant; particularly to his progress though treatment, and later recovery. The benefits of laughter have been generally accepted, especially in its effect on the release of pent up pressure. It releases endorphins in the brain that naturally tend to ease pain, and built up pressure. Humour plays a stress-moderating role. Much research has been done into the benefit of humour and its correlations to health and wellbeing. Freud (1905d) regarded humour as the highest of the defensive processes (a defence mechanism), and that humour provided a savings of emotional energy. The essence of it is that one protects oneself from affects that would have naturally arisen, during a stressful situation, by overriding the affect, and emotional reaction, with humour. This is a beneficial process due to its liberating elements signifying the triumph not only of the ego, but also of the pleasure principle, which is strong enough to assert itself here in the face of the adverse real circumstances. Martin and Lefcourt (1983) state:

> [E]nthusiastic acclamations of humor as a healthful coping strategy have been expressed by a number of theorists since Freud. Allport (1950), for example, states that "the neurotic who learns to laugh at

himself may be on the way to self-management, perhaps to cure" (p. 92). Rollo May (1953) states that humor has the function of "preserving the sense of self [...] It is the healthy way of feeling a 'distance' between one's self and the problem, a way of standing off and looking at one's problem with perspective. (p. 61) (p. 1314)

B indeed made use of this "defence mechanism" and may have very well been a coping strategy that helped him on the way to "self-management" and success.

Historical background

B stated that up until he was about four years old his parents seemed to be happy and he felt loved. In spite of the history, he has a good relationship with each parent. However, when he was about four years old things began to change as his parents begun to have a traumatic, emotionally abusive relationship. They eventually got divorced when he was twelve. His mother had suffered a slight breakdown during and after the divorce, and had gone through a period of depression, and had attempted to take her own life several times. He expressed that his mother did her best, but was not able to overcome the emotional abuse from his father. He stated that he wished that she had left his father earlier to avoid the trauma, and near self-destruction, of what she had been through. B stated that watching his mother go through this caused him the greatest anguish accompanied by feelings of fear of losing her and complete helplessness.

B stated that during the twelve years that his parents were together he had wished that they would break up. He felt that he went through his early life being a *passive* victim of his parents' abusive relationship, and experiencing feelings of extreme anxiety. He likened this to being a victim of "second-hand smoke".

He related that there were times when all he wanted to do was to run away, to escape all of the fighting. In an effort to "escape" he had invented a game that he would play (by himself). It was "an imagination game" that was like "a game of chess in the sky with live monsters". He was able to control the "pawns" and in this way he would create an "escape to another world to get away" from the trauma of his parents' fights.

The fantasy game

This was clearly an effort on B's part to escape the intensely traumatic situation. At four years old, he felt forgotten and abandoned, while his parents fought. There was a grave sense of vulnerability, and he had no one to protect him from what he saw and heard. He remembered being terrified.

The "fantasy chess game" is significant in the analysis, as it seemed to be his effort to objectify his pain and to have a sense of control over his situation. It was also, I suggest, a precursor to the self-destructive use of drugs to escape his past and to ease his anxieties. It was a way of soothing and comforting himself. It was as if he had created this game out of his emotional trauma where he took his pain and transformed it into a game and set it outside of himself. In separating himself from it as such, he was able to control its various aspects and in this way, he was safe.

In the safety of his mind, he endeavoured to gain some level of control over his situation. The game consisted of two teams of monsters. The monsters were like the pieces of a game of chess that he controlled and moved. Each pawn represented a person in his life and he "moved" them according to his rules placing the monsters in whatever strategic position he chose and moved them accordingly. He was the master in this fantasy and was bigger than these monsters, and the sense of omnipotence was significant to his survival.

He controlled his environment and preserved his existence in this space that was only known to him. Dodes (1990) states that the ability to be "powerful over oneself and one's internal state may also be described as an inherent aspect of narcissism. [...] among the strands of narcissism is the pleasure in efficient mental functioning, [...] the regulation of mood [...] and [...] a sense of inner safety and reliability" (p. 400).

This was apparent in B's creation of the fantasy game, which he returned to every time he was faced with an external situation, namely that of his parents fighting and the fear and anger that he experienced, which he could not control.

B stated that he was not able to speak about this fantasy before, as it seemed like "something weird" that he could not explain. However, on the other hand he stated that he was quite impressed with himself for creating this game and it was a space in his head where he could escape to. During his discussion about this fantasy, B came upon the idea that the drugs were a substitute for this game. Since the game was a tool that he used when he was much younger the drugs, now, were a "progression" to the next level.

The drug use was a "real" way to take revenge on those who had put him in the position to want to escape. It was a way of saying, "To hell with you, I'll do what I please." During our discussions, B expressed that using drugs was a way of releasing his anger and aggression and feeling out of control and at the same time it was a reparative effort to regain control and mastery.

Dodes (1990) further explains the significance of a "steadily regulable, containable affect for the development and organization of self-experience, without which affects become traumatic. [...] the narcissistic importance of being in control of one's mind. [...] a person may become enraged because he is suddenly not in control of his own thought processes, of a function which [we] consider to [...] [belong] to the core of our self, and we refuse to admit that we may not be in control of [it]" (ibid., p. 400).

B expressed a sense of rage at himself for feeling powerless and vulnerable to humiliation, loss, and rejection. There was also rage at his parents, namely his mother, for not protecting him against these feelings. His need to be in control was apparent throughout his discussion. He refused to admit defeat and said so in so many words.

He giggled at the most serious points during his sessions. It seemed to be an effort to waylay any risk of losing control. There were periods of time when he would dismiss any fear of demise. Freud's (1927d) theory on humour may be applied to this scenario:

> The grandeur in it clearly lies in the triumph of narcissism, the victorious assertion of the ego's invulnerability. The ego refuses to be distressed by the provocations of reality, to let itself be compelled to suffer. It insists that it cannot be affected by the traumas of the external world; it shows, in fact, that such traumas are no more than occasions for it to gain pleasure. (p. 163)

B saw his mother sink further and further into insecurity, losing her confidence and becoming depressed. He recalled how his mother stammered and stated, towards the end of our sessions, that his mother had not stammered for many years and he thinks that it was because she gradually, over the years, was able to "get away from all the abuse" and live her own life.

He said that he wanted to help, but he felt helpless. He expressed that, from time to time, he is aware that he will also stammer in the middle of a stressful conversation, and that his life at the present was like a period of "stammering"—where he was stuck and felt confused as to how to go on. It was like trying to get a certain word out and being stuck at the beginning of it in the stammer.

His mother's distress overwhelmed him. The periods when he stammered, he felt as if he was imitating his mother in an effort to know how to help her—as if he identified with her somehow. However, the sense of inadequacy that he felt caused him to stammer even more which made him frustrated and afraid of being humiliated. His desire to have control over his life was as great as his feelings of powerlessness. During the session where he related this, he began to stammer. He would stop speaking and point out that he was stammering. He would then giggle and joke about it for a few minutes. It seemed that at these times he needed to take a break from the intensity of his conversation. He would laugh to relieve his tension and regain his composure.

B stated that it hurt him to see his mother in so much pain. He speculated that his mother was affected by the experiences of rejection from her own family as well as her marriage, that it seemed as if she could not think for herself and had no power over her own life and circumstances. He developed a resentment towards his other family members and expressed that he even resented his mother for not standing up for herself. He resented her weakness because he felt that he had to look after her and was not able to do so.

He felt that he was robbed of a free and happy childhood and did not wish to be so powerless and to be controlled by others. It was clear that from the age of four to about twelve his expectations of his parents, especially of his mother, became frustrated and he felt let down and his hopes shattered.

The trauma of his mother's second marriage brought back fears and anxiety of his past. He struggled in school and eventually left without completing his grades to his mother's dismay but, at that point, he did not want to care. He felt betrayed. He felt mistrusted regardless of his efforts. He felt as if he was "nowhere and going nowhere" and that there was no point in worrying about "doing the right thing" anymore. He did not care and just wanted to escape from his reality.

Here it seems that what Wurmser (1974) stated seems consistent with what was occurring in B's life at this time:

> [W]e find an emotional illness brewing independently, whether the drug enters or not. The specificity for its outbreak in manifest form lies in an experience of overwhelming crisis, accompanied by intense emotions like disillusionment and rage, depression, or anxiety, in an actualization of a lifelong massive conflict about omnipotence and grandiosity, meaning and trust—what we have just described as a narcissistic conflict. This actualization inevitably leads to massive emotional disruption and thus to the addictive search. (p. 825)

B quit school determined to work and be independent. He left his mother's home and moved a number of times between relatives until they discovered that he was smoking marijuana. They told him that they would not tolerate these kinds of activities.

Shortly thereafter, B moved back in with his father. He said that his father did not seem to be interested in him or in what he was doing. He felt, increasingly, as if he did not belong to anyone or anywhere. He became involved with weight lifting and this activity brought him a sense of satisfaction. At the same time he realised that on the one hand, he was trying to keep fit and on the other hand, he was destroying what he was achieving due to his drug-taking activities, which also included the use of steroids.

B admitted that he had been using not only marijuana, but had also tried a number of other drugs including cocaine and ecstasy. In the last year, he had gone from working full time to giving up his job due to his circumstances, as a result of his drug use. B was out of work and money and this took him to the depths of depression where he started going to all-night dance clubs and the drug taking became a regular activity.

B stated that he worked odd jobs to maintain his drug habit. His doctor had diagnosed him with hypertension and high blood pressure. He admitted that he knew that he was destroying his body and wanted to stop doing what he was doing. However, being high was his only release from his thoughts and his life. He felt that he had no direction in life. He had nothing to talk about with anyone, family especially, so he avoided seeing them. He stated that his life felt empty and many a time he had asked himself, "Is this it?" and "Is this all that life is about—nothingness?" B stated that he did not know what he wanted and where he wanted to go. He had tried to quit using drugs, but he felt that his thoughts haunted him and the emptiness was unbearable.

He felt guilty, embarrassed, and confused about what had happened to his family and felt powerless to fix any of it. At the same time, he felt "forgotten". It seemed clear at this point that B was using drugs as an attempt at self-medication. As Wurmser stated, the importance of the effect of the drugs "in the inner life of these patients can perhaps be best explained as an artificial or surrogate defense against overwhelming affects" (1974, p. 828).

Freud (1930a) also described drugs as a means of coping with pain and disillusionment. As B stated, he still felt empty and lonely when he was taking drugs, but at least it did not seem to matter as much.

The dream

B also talked about a recurring dream that he had had during his teens especially when he started using drugs daily. He had some-times thought about it and it made him afraid. He could not figure out why his thoughts kept returning to it: He said that he dreamt of what appeared to be a gathering at a funeral hall. It was a large room filled with people dressed in black and many of them crying quietly. He said that, in his dream, he tries to get through the crowd to see who it was. No one seemed to notice him. He finally pushed through the crowd and saw a coffin. He stopped and was afraid to go any further. When asked why, he stated that he was afraid because he knew that the person in the coffin was him.

B's mental suffering and his fear of being lost and ignored are promi-nent elements in his dream. He stated that he, actually, did not want to be noticed "like this", because he was embarrassed of his life. He knew better and felt guilty for going against his values. He felt as if he was dead to the "normal world" and no one noticed him, which is what he felt in reality.

He had isolated or "separated himself" from people who loved him and cared for him. He was alone, even in the room full of people, in his dream. He was afraid of the coffin, which represented his fear of being powerless over a sense of total annihilation. What he feared most is that seeing himself dead in his dream may have meant that that is what he really desired. He did want to escape, but not to die. Within all of this fear there was, at the same time, a perverse (almost sadistic) sense of satisfaction in knowing that those who had caused him to have a "tragic life" would now grieve *their* loss. It was a kind of vengeance.

Here, as in the fantasy game, it seems as if the dream was a vehicle to gaining a sense of control over his pain. B was caught up in compulsive drug use that was, clearly, a manifestation of his mental suffering and pain. In its recurring nature, it seemed to be a deliberate repetition by his unconscious to gain a sense of omnipotence over his life. As in the fantasy game, the dream was his endeavour to objectify his pain and to control it.

He stated that he sought pleasure from his drug use and his rationale was that he deserved to feel pleasure by any means. He, however, felt alone and caught up in a vicious cycle that perpetuated this behaviour and a "compulsion to repeat".

It seemed that his wish to master his deep emotional suffering was fulfilled by the pleasurable effect achieved by the drugs. On the other hand, the guilt and shame of his behaviour seemed to be "punishment" for this very behaviour. The coffin, in a way also represented the womb. He felt he had disappointed his mother, but she had also disappointed him. The other side of the sword was that he wanted to take revenge on her for not preventing his life of suffering and for emotionally abandoning him.

It was interesting that even though B was involved, heavily at times, in drug taking behaviour, he was also obsessed with his image. He never missed a day at the gym. He explained that lifting the heavy weights was painful, especially, when he had lost a lot of his body weight due to drugs. In spite of this he never stopped. The pain of guilt and punishment were all wrapped up in this "system" of his to survive and overcome the instability of the reality of his life.

B stated that when he felt the pain of his muscles being "ripped" there was also a sense of pleasure and satisfaction. He was focused on the sensations of his body and his mind looking only for instant gratification. Loose (2002) quotes Rado who explained that "[D]rugs provide a kind of satisfaction that by-pass the erotogenic zones. In that passing movement it avoids the complications inherent in the sexual usages of these zones. Addiction so to speak, sexualises the whole body, providing it with, what Rado called, an 'alimentary orgasm'" (p. 103).

B was clearly insightful about his life and his behaviour and expressed a desire to make changes so that he could "clean himself and his life up". When asked what the reasons were for him to use drugs he stated that it gives him what he needs, which is not only escape but also the pleasure of the escape. But, the pleasure soon becomes pain and that is when he becomes depressed and looks for another opportunity to escape. The "cause" of the addiction was a desire for pleasure and the "effect" of it was desire for more pleasure. Loose (2002) states: "Addiction incarnates the essence of the psychoanalytic symptom. Addiction incarnates—and openly demonstrates—the beyond of pleasure that is contained within the symptom; a beyond to which the subject is profoundly attached" (p. 110).

It was clear that the pain which B was suffering came from what was buried in his unconscious. His sense of fear of losing control and appearing weak and powerless was always at the forefront of his presentation. In many drug users, I have observed a sense of fear in their *own* behaviour. And, any discussion veering close to the seriousness of their drug use and the social and health dangers would set them on a track of trying to minimise the risks of what they were doing. B, in a similar fashion, would begin to giggle, or laugh out loud, at something that was said in the session.

He spent a whole session speaking about the dream and its contents and his own interpretations of it and why he was having the dream. It was not possible to delve into an analysis of the dream. However, because it seemed to affect such an emotional response in the client, it has been mentioned here. In one stance, it seemed to serve a similar purpose as his giggling did, which was to objectify his pain and to separate himself from the reality of his situation.

B stated that the dream may have been an extension of his fantasy game. The only difference is that in his fantasy game he felt in complete control because he was awake, and in the dream, he felt a lack of control because he was asleep. He stated that there was a sense of anxiety of not knowing whether or not he would suddenly disappear into "thin air". He stated that his anxiety was so great at times that it prevented him from sleeping.

It is quite clear to trace the pain that developed in B's life. He felt lost and empty; ashamed of his life as he admitted that no one close to him, that he knew, came from a "broken home". They were "normal" and he came from an "abnormal and dysfunctional family", but he said that he had no idea how to be "normal". So much so, that it seemed easy to "get wrapped up with the bad crowd". When he was "high", it did not matter and he seemed to fit in. But this did not last long.

Interestingly enough he said at one point that he felt that he deserved to feel good. And since all his life he had felt "bad" he was going to do whatever it took to feel good and to escape his problems.

The impact of B's traumatic experiences, with his parents, as a young child had impacted his sense of security, existence, and identity. B stated that he felt "lost and empty" and that he was "no one" and "going nowhere". The pain of his mental suffering became a part of his existence that he wanted to escape. There was the unconscious emotional trauma of loss and rejection and a sense of worthlessness.

More significantly, I propose that the existence of his relationship with his suffering or being in pain was that of a sense of "being owed" something from life which had dealt him an unfair deal. It was a determination to make pleasure out of his pain (to use his pain) to fulfil his desires to fill the void. There is a clear sense of loss of the first object of his desire (his mother) and his guilt and shame at not being able to "fix things". At the same time, he was in a desperate search for independence not only from his mother, but also from memories of his past painful experiences of abandonment.

His fixation was on fulfilling his desire which was filling the emptiness or void within his psychic functioning. His search was obvious in his explanation as were the pain of loss and fear of annihilation. Even though he "hung around with the wrong crowd", he was alone. His drugs were his "friends". His drug taking was in isolation as was the pleasure that he derived from it. He did not need anyone, as he had said, "I did not need anyone to make me feel bad any more". Therefore, he separated himself from any meaningful relationships.

> The encounter with others always implies an element of risk, of anxiety and, above all, of unpredictability. To be part of human culture and to take part in the social bond also implies that there is a price to pay. This price is the loss of total pleasure when castration cuts the child out of the unity with the mother and replaces it with an ordinary or limited kind of pleasure. Addiction creates the illusion that this total pleasure is attainable again. (Loose, 2006, p. 32)

The perversion of drug taking behaviour "indicates the search for a sexual satisfaction that belongs to an earlier stage of infantile sexual development". This is the oral stage and "addiction being a kind of oral perversion". Drugs can provide the instant gratification of infantile sexual wishes (ibid., p. 101). I agree with Loose in that when faced with frustration the addict will reach for the drug that will instantly gratify his needs. It is psychic pain that seems to cause and perpetuate drug taking behaviour.

The depression and anxiety of guilt, shame, and emptiness, as in the case of B are clearly elements that triggered repeated drug use. However, in B's case it is this psychic pain and mental suffering that created a fear of annihilation within him. Not only the pain of suffering, but also the pain of fear and anxiety, of the unknown, that seemed to motivate him to seek help and to make changes in his life.

B had stated that he knew that his drug taking was a rebellious action, but he deserved to feel good. He felt sorry for his mother and his father, but it was not up to him to solve their problems—he was the child and deserved to have "normal parents". He did not care about them anymore and wanted only to get his own life straightened out, but he would do this on his own terms and no one was going to tell him otherwise. His sense of humour and ability to laugh at himself and giggle (uncontrollably) at times seemed to work as a mechanism that helped him to separate himself from his pain in such a way in which he was able to control it. He was able to understand it thus and learn to manage it to, eventually, reach a drug free lifestyle. It was a struggle that he took on board with an obsession to succeed.

Conclusion

There are several theories on the causes of drug addiction and we have examined only a sample of them in this chapter. The search for the real roots of addiction and its cure is an ongoing endeavour. A cure for addiction is not possible unless the emotional pain is faced. There are as many varieties of causes for addiction, as there are individuals, and the influence and impact of their particular psychological, biological, environmental, and behavioural elements figure prominently in their subjective experiences.

The dynamics of addictions run as deep and wide as the workings of the human mind, body, and brain. The very concept of the unconscious and what is brought into it, or what our minds allow to be brought into consciousness adds to the multidimensional complexities of a problem like addiction.

To underscore the arguments in this book, addiction is a state of chronic pain—impacted by either indulgence or deprivation—imposed on the body. It invokes a sense of being alienated from the external world. It is a neurosis that stems from the conflicts of unconscious, sexual desires, emotional, mental suffering, and pain. Self-destructive, repetitive compulsive behaviour such as drug abuse, and other forms of self-harm such as, deprivation, as in anorexia nervosa, are expressions of this suffering, as are other types of chronic pain.

Addictive behaviour is conducted in isolation. There is no trust in the other to bring satisfaction, as it is the other (the first object of desire—the mother) that has caused the subject to be in a state of constant craving.

Pain becomes the object of desire for the subject. Unless there is a state of pain the state of pleasure is a vague and ambiguous idea. However, within this simple deduction there are the deep complexities of the desire for self-preservation that bring with it the unconscious emotions of fear, guilt, shame and revenge manifested in feelings of isolation, rejection, loss, aggression and abandonment and of being out of control and powerless.

Is the addiction the "symptom" defined psychoanalytically as a "solution for underlying conflict"—or is it the "chronic pain" that is the symptom? Loose (2006) in his description of a symptom states:

> [T]he symptom is a solution to an underlying conflict. This defini-
> tion, of course, implies that the solution is not perfect: it does not
> resolve anything. The symptom is only a symptom in so far as it is
> repeated. If subjects repeat symptoms, there must be something in
> the symptom that the subject does not want to let go of, despite the
> fact that it causes suffering. This is precisely the issue that Freud
> tried to resolve with his theoretical concept of the death-drive.
> (p. 109)

Pain is expressed in a variety of ailments such as withdrawal and the management of depression, anxiety, paranoia, abuse, trauma, grief and immense cravings that need to be addressed, along with diseases of the liver, lungs and joints. There are also external conflicts of family, rela-tionships, and financial complications. Addiction is, on the one hand, a *solution* against unconscious suffering and, on the other hand, a *defence mechanism* that creates the pain which is needed to sustain that defence. Pain is, therefore the desired object and the symptom. It is the pain that the subject does not want to let go of. Addictive behaviour gives rise to a world of fantasy where pain is overcome by the dominance of pleasure. Here pain (unconscious mental suffering and its manifest behaviours) is manipulated to achieve pleasure.

Addictive behaviour allows the subject to escape into a narcissistic realm of self-preservation and a blurred state of constant pain and pleasure. It is his compulsion to repeat that which he believes he can control—in order to gain mastery over his pain. Thus he continues to repress his internal suffering and conflict setting up his defences in addictive, self-destructive behaviour perpetuating his fantasy of omnipotence, revenge and dominance over his loss and the object that caused his loss.

Dodes (1990) states that it is essential to consider the role of addiction in managing omnipotence over one's own affective state:

> The central importance of being in control of one's affective state is highlighted by the loss of this control in psychic trauma: i.e., the imposition of a state of helplessness on the ego when it is overwhelmed by an instinctual drive (affect) which it cannot manage without excessive anxiety (Freud, 1926). It is the sense of powerlessness or helplessness in this situation which [...] constitutes the essence of psychic trauma. (pp. 399–400)

Whether the addiction is indulgence in mind altering drugs or deprivation, underlying emotional trauma lies at the heart of the cause. The subject's life revolves around this chronic emotional pain that is manifested within behaviours such as repetitive self-harm.

The metaphor of the phantom can be applied here, as well. There is a profound sense of loss within the addicted subject. It is a loss a kin to the loss of a limb. He tries to fill the void with his behaviour only to perpetuate pain within the space. The neurosignatures (and the *psychosignatures*) attempt to repair the breach, as in the case of an amputation; the only difference is that the whole body is experiencing a physical as well as a psychological and emotional *non-existence* or *fragmented* "whole". On the one hand, the signatures attempt to find what is missing and to repress the loss, and on the other hand they try to compensate for it.

Neurobiology and psychology, of course work in tandem and the two must meet somewhere however, as Freud found in his 1895 *Project* (1950a) that not all psychological pain and suffering can be explained away through "scientific" evidence. Nevertheless, it gives us a wider perspective and a place to begin to understand the complexities of human behaviour, which I argue, is contingent upon the subject's relationship with his pain and, in turn, impacts his identity and existence.

CONCLUSION

Throughout this book, I have endeavoured to put together a mosaic of perspectives from which to begin to formulate a response to my curiosity—as well as my concern from a clinical perspective—regarding a more effective framework for viewing the painful issues which my clients bring into the counselling arena. I would like to endeavour to draw together the various dimensions of my discussions throughout this book in order to establish feasibility for my proposal which states that the subject has a relationship with his pain, and that this relationship impacts his identity and existence.

Pain is a topic which has been thought about, debated, and discussed throughout history (Rey, 1995; Dormandy, 2006). Schopenhauer (1969) has summarised the cause of this in saying that as long as we desire that which we lack, this desire exceeds the value of all other things in life until it is fulfilled. However, once what is desired is acquired it loses its value, appearing to be something different than what was expected and "a similar longing always holds us fast, as we thirst and hanker after life" (Vol. I, p. 318).

He stated that we shut our eyes to the truth, that suffering is essential to life, as if it is a bitter medicine. We do not wish to know that suffering is something which we carry around within us as a perpetual internal spring and that it is not something which is external. However, we insist on seeking a particular, external source or cause as if it will vindicate the pain that is always with us. He compares this state of human desire to "the free man" who "makes for himself an idol, in order to have a master" (ibid.). An example, from the *Book of Exodus* (32:1–30) is of the plight of the Israelites from Egypt which brought to each his own pain of loss and desire. They created something that they could see, touch, feel, and control. "God" had brought them what they desired. However, in receiving this, the pain of *captivity* returned as they were once again controlled by their desires. Schopenhauer goes on to say that "we untiringly strive from desire to desire, and although every attained satisfaction, however much it promised, does not really satisfy us, but often stands before us as a mortifying error" (ibid.).

Freud (1924b, 1925e) was influenced by Schopenhauer as he was by others which figure in the width and depth of his work from *A Project for a Scientific Psychology* (1950a) to *The Interpretation of Dreams* (1900a), and *Beyond the Pleasure Principle* (1920g). He writes about pain that is rooted in desire due to object loss and adheres to Schopenhauer's theory that desire precedes every pleasure, but that in satisfaction desire as well as pleasure ceases:

> [W]hen everything is finally overcome and attained, nothing can ever be gained but deliverance from some suffering or desire; consequently, we are only in the same position as we were before this suffering or desire appeared. What is immediately given to us is always only the want, i.e., the pain. (Schopenhauer, 1969, Vol. I, p. 319)

Pain is on our minds, in our hearts and in our lives. If it were not for pain, we would not be curious about pleasure. If desire and satisfaction impact the most essential dimensions of human existence—pleasure and pain—my argument then, that the subject has a relationship with his pain which, in turn, impacts his sense of identity and existence, is viable. The aspect of *relationship* is the key component to adhere to when considering psychological and emotional pain, as it is the relationship between the individual's desire and what he desires—pain. Pain is the precedent to every pleasure.

Throughout my book I have discussed Freud's psychoanalytical theories, which I derived to be explored in his (1895) *Project* that primarily set out to investigate his neurological theory of pain and pain processing. In the same way I have also examined Melzack and Wall's gate control theory (which began in the 1960s) and Melzack's theory of the neuromatrix (in the 1990s), systems in the brain that modulate the experience of pain, and the consequent cognitive and behavioural processes.

The purpose of this exploration was to show that the research that Freud began in 1895, toward a "scientific psychology", was taken up by later scientists to evidence that first of all there is a significant correlation between neurobiological and psychological and emotional pain, secondly that psychological and emotional pain do not need to be derived from a physical or external impact and third, interestingly, that physical pain, inevitably, has a psychological and emotional component. Even in cases where sensitivity to pain is absent, this absence has an impact on the psychological and emotional systems of the mind. Morris (1993) gives an example of Edward Gibson, "the human pincushion", who, due to his lack of sensitivity to pain, took advantage of this to create a stage act that shocked and stunned audiences. He stuck pins and spikes into various parts of his body, even enacting the Crucifixion that brought great emotional pain to his audience. Morris stated that this insensitivity to pain proved, to Gibson, a meaningless benefit that left him "indifferent". Gibson could never really know what he was "missing". Even though he did not experience physical pain the way you or I feel, he seemed to live in a world of pain. This was a kind of anxiety of the unknown, and a desire to know himself, as a "whole", and his reason for existence. "He could never figure out how to turn his strange gift into something more than a spectacle" (p. 13).

This investigation was inspired by the evidence that the neurological system does not function independently of the psychological system. Freud identified from his project that emotional pain does not need to have an external basis or "peripheral" impact. Melzack and Wall's (1996) theory of the "neuromatrix" explains that this is a system in the brain, from within which is created a "neurosignature". The signature is created from innate and historical activities, and facilitates responses to events and experiences. Inputs from experiences modulate the neurosignature, but cannot generate a new signature. Our cognitive and behavioural responses are innately set. However, these are influenced and modulated by external as well as internal experiences. Similarly, Freud (1950a) discussed the impact of and the responses to internal and external stimuli, through the nervous system. He postulated that responses to the stimuli are facilitated by permeable and impermeable neurons. This process creates the environment that allows for the formation of memory, perception, and motives. This explains how we perceive our bodies as a whole integrative system.

What is significant to this book is Freud's meta-psychological postulations that there does not need to be an external cause for pain. The neuromatrix is an explanation for the neurobiology of pain but it includes an appreciation that this has an impact on the subject's psychology. It, however, speaks from the stance that pain is a physical experience influenced by neurological and biological factors that can impact one's psychological state of mind.

My argument that there is a parallel development of a "psychomatrix" is, of course, derived from the notion of the neuromatrix. However, I propose that this is a matrix that does not exist in the brain but in the mind. The unconscious is the matrix within which there is an innate psychomatrix, and similar to the neuromatrix, impacts the perception of the "whole". The "whole" in this case, however, includes an essential sense of emotional wholeness that connects the body's dualism of phenomenal as well as psychological awareness and experience. It is this sense of emotional balance that is achieved by the reconciliations of our desire for the lost object and the fulfilment of that desire and its cycle of pain and pleasure. Within the psychomatrix is created an innate psychosignature that is modulated by and responds to our experiences of emotional pain. This is pain that is an anthology of our experiences that is imprinted in our unconscious mind. Freud (1900a, p. 578) clearly states that what has been imprinted in the unconscious, is never lost but comes to the surface under the influence of certain events and experiences.

What I have begun to explore within this book is the connection between what Freud started in the nineteenth century and what has been further understood and discovered later toward an understanding of the subject-pain relationship. His research has taken the science of psychology into the twenty-first century. I propose that in order to appreciate the nature of psychological and emotional pain, an investigation into the neurobiological nature of pain was essential. In order to answer my thesis question I needed to explore the science of psychology to begin to have a "whole" perspective on suffering as in *being in pain*. Pain that is "the precedent of every pleasure" and further that beyond the acquisition of pleasure is, again, pain (Schopenhauer, 1969, p. 319).

Therefore, it is essential to my argument to understand the aspects of the mind/body link identified throughout Freud's work, where he explains the dimensions of narcissism, repetition, and perversion which are key components to development.

Pertinent to an understanding of the processes of the body are other external influences that impact our sense of identity and existence, such as, religious and cultural beliefs, and the familial, social, and political environments that one lives within (Gibson, 1978; Scarry, 1985; Morris, 1993; Dormandy, 2006). Rey (1995) suggests "pain involves a codified form of social behaviour which sets the parameters of allowable overt manifestations and regulates the expression of such innermost personal experiences, whether endured in the family bosom or alone in a solitary confrontation with the self" (p. 5).

I have endeavoured to evidence that the subject-pain relationship impacts his identity and is a means to understanding how and why he relates, not only to himself, but also to others. Therefore, an exploration of how internal and external factors influence the subject's experience of pain, were part and parcel of this thesis. The knowledge that he is suffering impacts the subject's world view in how he views himself but, most importantly, how this impacts his relationship with others as well as himself, through suffering his pain. This, consequently, impacts his identity and the meaning of his existence in relation to his internal and external environment.

This book has strived to explore the subject-pain relationship through the psychoanalytic formulations on neurosis, perversion, narcissism, and loss. I examined the significance of how these internal mechanisms, of the unconscious and sexuality, impact on conscious manifestations, such as chronic pain syndrome, throughout an individual's life.

If Freud was right in his postulation regarding the desire of the subject, to re-find the object, could it not be that the subject needs to know his pain in such a way as to be able to know the direction in which he travels to fulfil his desire? To know his pain, then, would mean that he would know his pleasure, and the very presence of this aspect of human existence, in turn, begs a relationship with his pain.

According to Freud (1900a, 1920g, 1926), the most significant component within human development is a defence against the *dark* psychological and emotional experiences that make up "loss" and the desire for that which is lost. In the scenario of the phantom limb syndrome, we see the mechanisms at play that create a barrier to further trauma. The brain reorganises its "map" to compensate for the missing limb. It allows the body and the mind to accept the loss of the limb through a dichotomous experience of a phantom limb. The subject needs to be able to *feel* that he is still "whole" lest the emptiness, within the space that is left behind from the missing limb, overpowers his emotional integrity. The neurosignature, within the neuromatrix, is modulated by the experiences of the patient; however, it remains consistent in processing the response to this trauma so that the *physical sense* of "whole" remains intact (Melzack & Wall, 1996).

I proposed that a parallel process with the psychomatrix takes place. Once the acute event is stabilised it is not only the brain that goes to work, but more critically, it is the mind that must confront and comfort the emotional trauma of the subject. A *sense of being* "whole" impacts the subject's sense of identity. As is found in Freud's (1920g) theory of *the pleasure principle,* systems of the mind (and the brain) are guided by the "principle of constancy" or keeping the "excitation" in the "mental apparatus" down to as low a level as possible. The aim is to avoid unpleasure or stimulation over a certain limit (p. 9).

The phantom limb can also be used as a metaphor that can be applied to the example of other chronic pain as in fibromyalgia as well as addictions. It could also be applied to the biological lack of sensitivity to physical pain as the subject feels the *phantom* of that which is missing. Pain is caused by loss that in turn causes emotional trauma which is for the most part repressed in our unconscious, manifesting in a variety of forms throughout development. As these emotions make themselves known via memories within the conscious, provoking certain behaviour, it is clear that Freud regarded memory and motive to work in tandem. "Memories have no meaning or power unless they are allied with motives" (Solms, 1998, p. 19).

It is the power of memories that impacts the formation of subjective identity. However, because memories have great reconstructive powers they also have the potential to (re)construct identity and meaning of existence. Within the processes of memories, there is the primary motive which is to fulfil a desire for that which was lost. At the basis of this motive is not only loss by a need to avenge oneself from being subjected to trauma. Hence the concept of "screen memories" (Freud, 1905) that are a compromise between repressed elements and the defence against them.

It appears that the subject's relationship to pain is steeped in a need for power and control. This is a need to maintain the integrity of the "whole", which is an integration of the physical, psychological and emotional integrity of the "self". As previously stated in this book, "the phenomenology of self is so deep and intangible that it sometimes seems illusory" (Chalmers, 1997, p. 10). Pain brings to consciousness an orchestration of sensations that do not always "sound" harmonious to the unities of body, brain, and mind. However, within all of that there is the "background hum" of the experience of the self and its relationship with pain. The subject is conscious of his *relationship* as a "hum" that tells him that he exists and that he must somehow defend this existence. Not always in the sphere of the conscious, indeed the self is mostly unconscious, and as Freud (1923b) has expressed, what is conscious is only "the tip of the iceberg".

In Chapter One, I explored Freud's (1895) scientific research in his *Project*, as well as that of later scientists such as Melzack and Wall (1993, 1996, 2001) and others to show that the mechanisms of the body and the brain are influenced by, and according to, biologically embedded coding, and the endogenous development of processing mechanisms.

I have explored the theories that mapped the excitatory and inhibitory processes of memory and motive that are significant to the understanding of emotional and psychological pain. Melzack's (1993) neuromatrix evidences that the brain perceives the body as a certain "whole". Even when there is a "cut" or dismemberment, either from birth or caused during one's life, the brain's mechanism continues to perceive the body as a "whole", therefore behaving as if it is "whole" (p. 621). This phenomenon, I believe, is what figures into the notion of "mourning a loss". The neuromatrix allows the brain to do more than detect and analyse inputs as it generates perceptual experience even when no external inputs occur (p. 628).

These perceptual experiences also become part of the emotional dynamics of the development of the subject's relationship with pain, identification of self, and meaning of existence.

Through this investigation, I identified that there were physical as well as psychological processes at work. Some of these are conscious and some unconscious. The unconscious processes could be inferred by the conscious ones. Consciousness has two features, an external perception of the world and an internal perception of the inner workings of the mind which "represents the unconscious reality that lies within us in the form of subjective states of awareness—such as memories, beliefs, and desires" (Solms, 1998, p. 8).

Thus, the first key components in this thesis are the notions of memory and motive and the concept of the "whole" self. Memories are either activated or inhibited by a variety of processes, as explained by Freud's (1895) *Project*, Melzack and Wall's (1993, 1996, 2001) gate control theory, and Melzack's (1996) theory of the neuromatrix. The motive for these is human progression through the complexities of the stages of development. Experiences are imprinted on the mappings of the brain as well as the unconscious and are selectively accessed to allow certain cognitive and behavioural functioning.

The metaphor of the "gate" in Melzack and Wall's (1993) gate control theory is a modulation of the intensity of impacts of stimuli on the responses of the body and brain, for example sensory pain from a stubbed toe. This can be compared to the ego functioning of the mind as it modulates the materials (memories/experiences) in the mind and their impact on consciousness, for example repression and neurosis. Both impacts the conscious as well as the unconscious as memories of internal as well as external experiences become imprinted within the processes of the brain as well as the mind.

An exploration of Freud's theory of pain, in Chapter Two, took me further through his concepts of the unconscious and the life and death instincts. I also examined the definitions of "subject", "self", "relationship", "identity", "existence", and "pain".

Chapters Three, Four, Five and Six were opportunities for me to apply these concepts to the scenarios of chronic pain as in the phantom limb syndrome, fibromyalgia, as well as within addictions. Primarily they were explorations of the processes of chronic pain. The conversion between psychological pain and physical pain was significant to comprehend a narcissistic to object cathexis, and the process of the mind, transforming an acute physical trauma into a psychological trauma, (Freud, 1926d; Gamsa, 1994). Physical and psychological traumas trigger each other, as in the opponent process theory (Solomon, 1980). Repetition of past trauma are the reactions of the mind and body matrices—that in turn trigger the emotional state of "being in pain" as opposed to "having pain" (Pontalis, 1981).

Following what has already been expressed, I believe that it is important to also understand that Freud conceived that the truth of reality was influenced by our subjective perceptions, which flow from our unconscious and which distort or even filter the truth of reality. Therefore, my definition of pain as a conglomerate is necessary for then, it is irrelevant whether or not a memory has been distorted. What is significant is that the *feeling* experience of a past trauma continues to exist. The reality is that the subject experiences *being in pain* which is essential to his existence. The development of a relationship with pain is inevitable as it creates the "motive" for the preservation of self.

Within the phenomenon of chronic pains, we see how pain can be objectified and used to either destroy or create a certain identity. This identity, negative or positive, can, then, influence the subject's sense of self and therefore, impacts his response to stimuli from the internal and external environments of his existence.

My theory is that this suffering becomes embedded in the unconscious as a subjective memory and influences identity, existence, and behaviour. As Solms (1998) states, "internal, subjective awareness is where our patients *locate the suffering* that they bring to us in psychoanalysis" (pp. 7–9).

My final conclusion is that *pain* becomes an *object*—the object of desire—which compels the subject to respond accordingly and consequently. An understanding of this relationship is crucial as it draws out the motives for behaviour which could in turn impact the paradigms of *pain management*. To ignore "negative" emotions—as in repression—cannot be beneficial as psychoanalysis has evidenced, for *knowing* them, I agree, is the only way forward toward good mental health—but this does not mean being pain *free*.

The truth that Freud evidenced throughout his work is that pain is who we are. If we take away pain we take away who we are, and that it is not humanly possible to take away or cut pain out of our existence. To be in pain is the most essential component to our survival as it not only fulfils our sexual instincts and desire, but is also a defence against unconscious, unresolved emotional trauma. We also need to be able to comprehend the objectification of pain in order to see it more clearly as something that can be mastered to achieve the pleasure that we seek.

REFERENCES

Aguirre, M. C. (2011). Bulimia, anxiety, and the demand of the other. In: Y. G. Baldwin, K. Malone, & T. Svolos (Eds.), *Lacan and Addiction: an Anthology* (pp. 177–185). London: Karnac.

American Psychiatric Association (2000). *Diagnostic and statistical manual of mental disorders* (4th ed., text rev.). Washington, DC: APA.

Ausubel, D. P. (1980). An interactional approach to narcotic addiction. In: D. J. Lettieri, M. Sayers, & H. W. Pearson (Eds.), *Theories on Drug Abuse: Selected Contemporary Perspective. NIDA Research Monograph 30* (pp. 4–8). Rockville, MD: National Institute on Drug Abuse. http.//archives. drugabuse.gov/pdf/monographs/download30.html [last accessed 27 April 2015].

Beckett, S. (1953). The Unnamable. New York (NY): Grove, 1958.

Bejerot, M. (1980). Addiction to pleasure: a biological and social-psychological theory of addiction. In: D. J. Lettieri, M. Sayers, & H. W. Pearson (Eds.), *Theories on Drug Abuse: Selected Contemporary Perspectives, NIDA Research Monograph 30* (pp. 246–255). Rockville, MD: National Institute on Drug Abuse.

Bokan, J., Ries, R. K., & Katon, W. J. (1981). Tertiary gain and chronic pain. *Pain, 10*: 331–335.

203

Bond, M. R., & Pearson, I. B. (1969). Psychological aspects of pain in women with advanced cancer of the cervix. *Journal of Psychosomatic Research, 13*: 13–39.

Bowlby, J. (1969). *Attachment and Loss, Vol. 1: Attachment*. New York, NY: Basic Books.

Bowlby, J. (1973). *Attachment and Loss, Vol. 1: Separation*, New York, NY: Basic Books

Bowlby, J. (1978). Attachment theory and its therapeutic implications. In: S. C. Feinstein & P. L. Giovacchini (Eds.), *Adolescent Psychiatry: Development and Clinical Studies* (pp. 5–23). Chicago, IL: University of Chicago Press.

Bozarth, M. A. (1994). Pleasure systems in the brain. In: D. M. Warburton (Ed.), *Pleasure: the Politics and the Reality* (pp. 5–14). New York, NY: Wiley.

Byck, R. (Ed.) (1974). *Cocaine Papers, Sigmund Freud*. New York, NY: Stonehill.

Carsten, E. (2009). Neurobiology of itch and pain: scratching for answers. In: J. Castro-Lopes (Ed.), *Current Topics in Pain: 12th World Congress on Pain* (pp. 73–93). Seattle, WA: IASP.

Centonze, D., Siracusano, A., Calabresi, P., & Bernardi, G. (2004). A project for a scientific psychology (1895): a Freudian anticipation of LTP-memory connection theory. *Brain Research Reviews, 46* (3): 310–314.

Cooper, A. M. (1991). The unconscious core of perversion. In: G. I. Fogel & W. A. Myers (Eds.), *Perversions and Near Perversions in Clinical Practice: New Psychoanalytic Perspectives* (pp. 17–35). New Haven, CT: Yale University Press.

Dansak, D. (1973). On the tertiary gain of illness. Journal of Comprehensive Psychiatry, *14* (6): 523–534.

Dodes, L. M. (1990). Addiction, helplessness, and narcissistic rage. *The Psychoanalytic Quarterly, 59*: 398–419.

Dormandy, T. (2006). *The Worst of Evils: the Fight against Pain*. New Haven, CT: Yale University Press.

Doyle, D. (Ed.) (2010). Obituaries. *Journal of The Royal College of Physicians of Edinburgh, 40*: 188. www.rcpe.ac.uk/journal/issue/journal_40_2/notable-fellows.pdf [last accessed 24 April 2015].

Engel, G. L. (1959). "Psychogenic" pain and the pain-prone patient. *American Journal of Medicine, 26* (6): 899–919.

Evans, D. (2005). *An Introductory Dictionary of Lacanian Psychoanalysis*. New York, NY: Routledge.

Felluga, D. (2011). Modules on Lacan: on psychosexual development. *Introductory Guide to Critical Theory*. www.cla.purdue.edu/english/theory/psychoanalysis/lacandevelop.html [last accessed 27 April 2015].

Finger, S., & Hustwit, M. P. (2003). Five early accounts of phantom limb in context: Pare, Descartes, Lemos, Bell, and Mitchell. *Neurosurgery, 52* (3): 675–686.

Freud, A. (1981). A psychoanalyst's view of sexual abuse by parents. In: P. B. Mrazek & C. H. Kempe (Eds.), *Sexually Abused Children and their Families* (pp. 33–34). Oxford: Pergamon.

Freud, S. (1891b). *On Aphasia*. London: Imago, 1953.

Freud, S. (1894a). The neuro-psychoses of defence. *S. E., 3*: 43. London: Hogarth.

Freud, S. (1895d). *Studies on Hysteria. S. E., 2*. London: Hogarth.

Freud, S. (1900a). *The Interpretation of Dreams. S. E., 4–5*. London: Hogarth.

Freud, S. (1905d). *Three Essays on the Theory of Sexuality. S. E., 7*: 125. London: Hogarth.

Freud, S. (1905e). Fragment of an analysis of a case of hysteria. *S. E., 7*: 3. London: Hogarth.

Freud, S. (1909d). Notes upon a case of obsessional neurosis. *S. E., 10*: 155. London: Hogarth.

Freud, S. (1913j). The claims of psycho-analysis to scientific interest. *S. E., 13*: 165. London: Hogarth.

Freud, S. (1914c). On narcissism: an introduction. *S. E., 14*: 69. London: Hogarth.

Freud, S. (1914g). Remembering, repeating and working-through (further recommendations on the technique of psycho-analysis, II). *S. E., 12*: 147. London: Hogarth.

Freud, S. (1916–1917). *Introductory Lectures on Psycho-Analysis. S. E., 15–16*. London: Hogarth.

Freud, S. (1917e). Mourning and Melancholia. *S. E., 14*: 239. London: Hogarth.

Freud, S. (1920g). *Beyond the Pleasure Principle. S. E., 18:* 7. London: Hogarth.

Freud, S. (1921c). *Group Psychology and the Analysis of the Ego. S. E., 18*: 69. London: Hogarth.

Freud, S. (1923b). *The Ego and the Id. S. E., 19*: 3. London: Hogarth.

Freud, S. (1924b). Neurosis and Psychosis. *S. E., 19*: 149. London: Hogarth.

Freud, S. (1924c). The Economic Problem Of Masochism. *S. E., 19*: 157. London: Hogarth.

Freud, S. (1924d). The Dissolution Of The Oedipus Complex. *S. E., 19*: 173. London: Hogarth.

Freud, S. (1925e). The Resistances To Psycho-Analysis. *S. E., 19*: 213. London: Hogarth.

Freud, S. (1926d). *Inhibitions, Symptoms and Anxiety. S. E., 20*: 77. London: Hogarth.

Freud, S. (1927d). Humour. *S. E., 21*: 159. London: Hogarth.

Freud, S. (1927e). Fetishism. *S. E., 21*: 149. London: Hogarth.

Freud, S. (1930a). *Civilization and its Discontents. S. E., 21*: 59. London: Hogarth.

Freud, S. (1933b). *Why War? S. E.*, 22: 197. London: Hogarth.

Freud, S. (1940a). *An Outline of Psycho-Analysis. S. E.*, 23: 141. London: Hogarth.

Freud, S. (1950a). A project for a scientific psychology. *S. E.*, 1: 175. London: Hogarth.

Freud, S. (1963). *The Cocaine Papers*. Vienna: Dunquin.

Fry, P. (2009). Jacques Lacan in theory. *Introduction to Theory of Literature*, Yale University lecture series (13), Department of English Literature.

Gamsa, A. (1993). The role of psychological factors in chronic pain. I. A half century of study. *IASP Journal of Pain, 57*: 5–15.

Gamsa, A. (1994). The role of psychological factors in chronic pain. II. A critical appraisal. *IASP Journal of Pain, 57*: 17–29.

Gibson, I. (1978). *The English Vice*. London: Duckworth.

Grey, W. (2000). Metaphor and meaning. *Minerva—An Internet Journal of Philosophy*, Volume 4 www.ul.ie/~philos/vol4/metaphor.html [last accessed 27 April 2015].

Hall, A. M., Kamper, S. J., Maher, C. G., Latimer, J., Ferreira, M. L., & Nicholas, M. K. (2011). Symptoms of depression and stress mediate the effect of pain on disability. *Pain, 152*: 1044–1050.

Halligan, P. W. (2002). Phantom limbs: the body in mind. *Cognitive Neuropsychiatry, 7* (3): 251–269.

Haythornthwaite, J. A. (2009). It's a belief. It's an appraisal. It's coping … No, it's catastrophizing. In: J. Castro-Lopes (Ed.), *Current Topics in Pain, 12th World Congress on Pain* (pp. 271–288). Seattle, WA: IASP.

Hong, V. H., & Hong, H. E. (Eds.) (2000). *The Essential Kierkegaard*. Princeton, NJ: Princeton University Press.

Huber, C., Kunz, M., Artelt, C., & Lautenbacher, S. (2010). Attentional and emotional mechanisms of pain and their related factors: a structural equations approach. *Journal of Pain Research and Management, 4*: 229–237.

Hughes, M., & Zimin, R. (1978). Children with psychogenic abdominal pain and their families. *Journal of Clinical Paediatrics, 17*: 569–573.

Jay, M. (2010). High Society: Mind-Altering Drugs in History and Culture. London: Thames & Hudson.

Joyce, P. A. (1995). Psychoanalytic theory, child sexual abuse and clinical social work. *Clinical Social Work Journal, 23* (2): 199–214.

Kaplan, L. J. (1991). Women masquerading as women. In: G. I. Fogel & W. A. Myers (Eds.), *Perversions and Near-Perversions in Clinical Practice: New Psychoanalytic Perspectives* (pp. 127–152). New Haven, CT: Yale University Press.

Khantzian, E. J., & Mack, J. E. (1983). Self-preservation and the care of the self—ego instincts reconsidered. *Psychoanalytic Study of the Child, 38*: 209–232.

Lacan, J. (1958). The direction of treatment and the principles of its power. In: B. Fink (Trans.) with H. Fink & R. Grigg, *Écrits: The First Complete Edition in English* (pp. 489–542). New York: Norton, 2006.

Lacan, J. (1977). *The Four Fundamental Concepts of Psycho-Analysis*. New York, NY: Norton.

Lacan, J. (1992). *The Seminar of Jacques Lacan Book VII: The Ethics of Psychoanalysis (1959–1960)*. New York, NY: Norton.

Lacan, J. (2003). Some reflections on the ego. In: A. C. Furman & S. T. Levy (Eds.), *Influential Papers from the 1950s, International Journal of Psychoanalysis Key Paper Series* (p. 298). London: Karnac.

Leshner, A. I. (1998). NIDA probes the elusive link between child abuse and later drug abuse. *NIDA Notes, 13* (2). http.//archives.drugabuse. gov/NIDA_Notes/NNVol13 N2/DirRepVol13 N2.html [last accessed 27 April 2015].

Lesse, S. (1974). Atypical facial pain of psychogenic origin: a masked depressive syndrome. In: S. Lesse, (Ed.), *Marked depression* (pp. 302–317). New York, NY: Jason Aronson.

Liebeskind, J. C. (1991). Pain can kill. *Pain, 44*: 3–4.

Loose, R. (2006). *The Subject of Addiction: Psychoanalysis and the Administration of Enjoyment*. London: Karnac.

Loose, R. (2007). *The Cause is the Effect*. [Unpublished article provided to inform my research on addiction and topic of his lecture at Brunel University.] DBS—Arts, Dublin.

Loose, R. (2011). Modern symptoms and their effects as forms of administration: a challenge to the concept of dual diagnosis and to treatment. In: Y. G. Baldwin, K. Malone, & T. Svolos (Eds.), *Lacan and Addiction: an Anthology* (pp. 1–37). London: Karnac.

Marrazzi, M. A., & Luby, E. D. (1986). An auto-addiction opioid model of chronic anorexia nervosa. *International Journal of Eating Disorders, 5* (2): 191–208.

Martin, R. A., & Lefcourt, H. M. (1983). Sense of humor as a moderator of the relation between stressors and moods. *Journal of Personality and Social Psychology, 45* (6): 1313–1324.

Melzack, R. (1993). Pain: past, present and future. *Canadian Journal of Experimental Psychology, 47* (4): 615–629.

Melzack, R. (2006). Phantom LIMBS. *Scientific American Special Edition, 16* (3): 52–59.

Melzack, R., & Wall, P. (1965). Pain mechanisms: a new theory. *Science, 3699*: 971–979.

Melzack, R., & Wall, P. D. (1996). *The Challenge of Pain*. London: Penguin.

Merskey, H. (1965). The characteristics of persistent pain in psychological illness. *Journal of Psychosomatic Research, 9*: 291–298.

Merskey, H. (1985). A mentalistic view of pain and behaviour. *Behaviour Brain Science, 8*: 65.

Merskey, H. (Ed.) (1986). Classification of chronic pain: descriptions of chronic pain syndromes and definitions of pain terms. *Pain, 3*: 226.

Merskey, H., & Boyd, D. (1978). Emotional adjustment and chronic pain. *Pain, 5*: 173–178.

Merskey, H., & Spear, F. G. (1967). *Pain: Psychological and Psychiatric Aspects.* London: Bailliere, Tindall & Cassell.

Mills, J. (2003). Lacan on paranoiac knowledge. *Psychoanalytic Psychology, 20* (1): 30–51.

Modell, A. H. (2003). Emotional memory, metaphor, and meaning. *Psychoanalytic Inquiry, 25* (4): 555–568. www.tandfonline.com/doi/abs/10.2513/s07351690pi2504_9# [last accessed 27 April 2015].

Morris, D. B. (1993). *The Culture of Pain.* Berkeley, CA: University of California Press.

Mularski, R. A., White-Chu, F., Overbay, D., Miller, L., Asch, S. M., & Ganzini, L. (2006). Measuring pain as the 5th vital sign does not improve quality of pain management. *Journal of General Internal Medicine, 21* (6): 607–612.

Nathanson, M. (1988). Phantom limbs as reported by S. Weir Mitchell. *Neurology, 38*: 504–505.

National Institute on Drug Abuse www.nida.nih.gov/ResearchReports/comorbidity/ [last accessed 2 March 2011]. NIDA Research Report Series (2010). pp. 1–12. (http.//www.nida.nih.gov/tib/comorbid.html, accessed 30 January 2011)

Parks, C. M. (1973). Factors determining the persistence of phantom pain in amputees. *Journal of Psychosomatic Research, 17*: 97–108.

Peele, S., & Alexander, B. K. (1998). *Theories of addiction. The Meaning of Addiction: An unconventional view.* San Francisco, CA: Jossey-Bass.

Pilowsky, I. (1994). Pain and illness behaviour: assessment and management. In: P. D. Wall & R. Melzack. R. (Eds.), *Textbook of Pain*, 3rd edn. (pp. 1309–1319). Edinburgh: Churchill Livingston.

Pontalis, J. B. (1981). *Frontiers in Psychoanalysis: Between the Dream and Psychic Pain.* London: Hogarth.

Pribram, K. H. (1962). The neuropsychology of Sigmund Freud. In: A. J. Bachrach (Ed.), *Experimental Foundations of Clinical Psychology* (pp. 442–468). New York, NY: Basic Books.

Pribram, K. H. (1998). A century of progress. In: R. M. Bilder & F. F. LeFever (Eds.), *Neuroscience of the Mind on the Centennial of Freud's Project for a Scientific Psychology* (pp. 11–19). New York, NY: New York Academy of Science.

Pribram, K. H., & Gill, M. (1976). *Freud's Project Reassessed.* London: Hutchinson.

Ramachandran, V. S. (1994). Phantom limbs, neglect syndromes, repressed memories, and Freudian psychology. *International Review of Neurobiology,* 37: 291–333.

Ramachandran, V. S., & Blakeslee, S. (1998). *Phantoms in the Brain, Probing the Mysteries of the Human Mind.* New York, NY: William Morrow.

Ramachandran, V. S., & Hirstein, W. (1998). The perception of phantom limbs. The D. O. Hebb lecture. *Brain, 121:* 1603–1630.

Rapaport, D. (1950a). *Emotion and Memory, 2nd edn.* New York, NY: International University Press.

Rey, R. (1995). *The History of Pain.* Cambridge, MA: Harvard University Press.

Sacks, O. W. (1998). Sigmund Freud: the other road. In: G. Guttmann & I. Scholz-Strasser (Eds.), *Freud and the Neurosciences, from Brain Research to the Unconscious* (pp. 11–22). Osterreichischen Akademie der Wissenschaften.

Schopenhauer, A. (1969). *The World as Will and Presentation, vol I.* New York, NY: Dove.

Schore, A. N. (2001). Minds in the making: attachment, the self-organizing brain, and developmentally-oriented psychoanalytic psychotherapy. *The British Journal of Psychotherapy, 17* (3): 299–328.

Solms, M. (1998). Before and after Freud's Project. In: R. M. Bilder & F. F. LeFever (Eds.), *Neuroscience of the Mind on the Centennial of Freud's Project for a Scientific Psychology* (pp. 1–10). New York, NY: New York Academy of Science.

Solomon, R. (1980). Opponent-process theory of acquired motivation: the costs of pleasure and the benefits of pain. *The American Psychologist, 35* (8): 691–712. www.psych.appstate.edu/~kms/classes/psy5150/Documents/Solomon1980_Opponent.pdf [last accessed 2 February 2011].

Spruiell, V. (1975). Three strands of narcissism. *Psychoanalytic Quarterly, 44* (4): 577–595.

Stanton, M. D. (1980). A family theory of drug abuse. In: D. J. Lettieri, M. Sayers, & H. W. Pearson (Eds.), *Theories on Drug Abuse: Selected Contemporary Perspective. NIDA Research Monograph 30* (pp. 147–155). Rockville, MD: National Institute on Drug Abuse. http.//archives.drugabuse.gov/pdf/monographs/download30.html [last accessed 20 January 2011].

Stoller, R. J. (1974). The hostility and mystery in perversion. *International Journal of Psychoanalysis, 55:* 425–434.

Stoller, R. J. (1991). The term perversion. In: G. I. Fogel & W. A. Myers (Eds.), *Perversions and Near-Perversions in Clinical Practice: New Psychoanalytic Perspectives* (pp. 36–56). New Haven, CT: Yale University Press.

Stoller, R. J. (2003). *Perversion: The Erotic Form of Hatred.* London: Karnac.

Swanson, D. W. (1984). Chronic pain as a third pathologic emotion. *American Journal of Psychiatry, 141:* 210–214.

Szasz, T. S. (1957). *Pain and Pleasure*. New York, NY: Basic Books.

Temple, L. K. F., McLeod, R. S., Gallinger, S., & Wright, J. G. (2001). Essays on science and society: defining disease in the genomics era. *Science, 293* (5531): 807–808.

Treurniet, N. (1991). Introduction to "On Narcissism". In: J. Sandler, E. S. Person, & P. Fonagy (Eds.), *Freud's "On Narcissism: An Introduction"* (pp. 75–94). New Haven, CT: Yale University Press.

University of Utah, Genetic Science Learning Centre (2006). Natural Reward Pathways Exist in the Brain. http.//learn.genetics.utah.edu/content/addiction/reward/ [last accessed 20 February 2011].

Violon, A. (1982). The process of becoming a chronic pain patient. In: R. Roy & E. Tunks (Eds.), *Psychosocial Factors in Rehabilitation* (pp. 20–35). London: Williams & Wilkins.

Wurmser, L. (1974). Psychoanalytic considerations of the etiology of compulsive drug use. *The Journal of the American Psychoanalytic Association,* 22: 820–843. www.cyberpsych.org/alcohol/wurmser.htm [last accessed 17 December 2010].

INDEX